KETO DIET FOR WOMEN OVER 50

THE ULTIMATE GUIDE TO KETO DIET FOR WEIGHT LOSS, WITH HEALTHY RECIPES FOR YOUR MEAL PREP. DISCOVER A UNIQUE 30-DAY MEAL PLAN.

DR. BRANDON HILL

TABLE OF CONTENTS

Introduction

The name "Keto" comes from the word "ketogenic" which refers to the metabolic state of ketosis that starts in the body when carbohydrate intake is suddenly reduced and replaced with healthy fats. Most people start a ketogenic diet to lose weight, not just in water weight but in abdominal and other stored fat. It resembles the Atkins and other low-carb diets. The primary guideline is to drastically reduce your consumption of carbohydrates and replace it with healthy fats. This dramatic reduction in carbohydrates helps your body enter a metabolic state called ketosis in which your body burns fat for fuel rather than glucose.

The average person eats foods loaded in carbohydrates, the liver then converts glucose. Your body creates insulin in order to move the glucose into the bloodstream, which distributes it throughout your body and brain. The body's primary source of energy is glucose whenever carbohydrates are present in the body. Your body will always use glucose over fat or any other energy source.

The keto diet is focused on not using glucose as your energy source but instead fat. Once your body enters ketosis, your body becomes effective at burning fat, losing weight and overall improving health. It also converts fat into ketones inside your liver, which can supply energy for the brain. The ketogenic diet can cause also cause a massive reduction in blood sugar and insulin levels.

Sometimes it can be difficult to detect whether or not you have entered ketosis. Here are several signs and symptoms that indicate you are in ketosis.

- Bad breath, most people have a smelly breath once they are fully into ketosis.

- Weight loss, most people expect rapid weight loss during the first week of the keto diet.

- Fatigue or excessive tiredness is a common sign of the keto flu.

- Extreme thirst and dehydration

- Use a urine test strip to measure your ketone levels

- Use a cheap ketone breathalyzer to detect how much ketones are in your blood

- Appetite suppression, most of the time you won't feel hungry when you enter ketosis

- *Digestive issues such as stomach pains, diarrhea, constipation and aches*

The keto diet or the ketogenic diet requires you to follow a meal plan that is low in carbs and high in fat. It has some similarities with diet plans like the Atkin's diet and other low-carb meal plans. The goal of this diet is to increase the fat content in the body and reducing the carbohydrate content to push your body into the ketosis state which turns you into a fat burning machine.

Benefits of ketogenic diet

Keto diet gets popular as it's a very effective way of weight loss, but research also shows that it doesn't only help you lose weight but also benefits your health greatly. When you use fat as fuel, your body becomes much active and sustainable. The extra energy will help you do workouts and improve your stamina.

The benefits which women can get from Keto diet are:

Energy level rise

Women after 50 don't have the same level of energy as 30 years women have. They struggle on doing the workout, but Keto has gotten your back. It helps in raising your energy level, so you don't feel bad about being weak. In the first days, you may feel so exhausted, tired but with the time your energy level rises and gives you strength, and your mind also works best with proper focus on the tasks you do.

Anxiety and depression diminish

The Keto diet also helps in reducing anxiety. This is due to the high intake of fat and a low level of sugar. A recent study also showed that the women who were on a Keto diet were not facing through anxiety and depression, but those who were not having this diet were more prone to depression.

Protection against Type 2 diabetes

The Keto diet also cut your sugar intake to less than 20g, and it helps in maintaining your blood sugar level if you are a diabetes patient. The type 2 patients also manage to control their blood sugar when putting into the Keto diet. This is very beneficial for women who have diabetes, and they are struggling with their weight as well.

Healthy body and lifestyle

Your life gets healthier when you are on a keto diet. Your intake of fat becomes more, and you consume very less sugar and carbs. The keto diet also helps to reduce fatty liver disease and other inflammation, which occurs due to eating more sweeteners and an unhealthy diet. Your body becomes fit, and you start living a healthy lifestyle.

Sound sleep time

Women who are on a Keto diet tell that they feel much satisfied and sound while sleeping, and their sleep cycle also improves drastically. Although in the first days you feel restlessness and tiredness with insomnia after 4-5 days, your sleep cycle gets better, and you would sleep longer, relaxed, and fulfilled when you wake up.

Keto diet may help in the treatment of cancer

Keto diet is also a way to treat very serious diseases, and cancer is one of them. It stops the growth of the tumor. The research showed that the ketones bodies may provide energy to your body without being the food for the cancerous tumor.

Cravings diminish

The benefit of a Keto diet is that you become habitual of the lifestyle you follow during this diet. You start controlling your blood sugar level, which helps in controlling cravings. You also feel that you can go long without having sweets or sugar. Intermitted fasting becomes common among women who have been on a Keto diet, which is very useful for your body.

Keto can improve your heart health and sharpen your brain

It may look strange that a diet filled with fats is beneficial for the heart, but it is true. In one year's study, 22 out of 26 cases of cardiovascular showed an improvement in their health conditions. Notably, these women experienced a Keto diet and intermittent fasting. Your brain also sharpens when you are on a Keto diet; there is a lot of evidence which are showing how significant this diet is. The brain works more efficiently on ketones than blood sugar. When you are on a normal diet, the brain gets 100% energy from glucose, but when you are on the keto diet, up to two-thirds of brain energy comes from ketones.

Improve chances of conceiving

Keto diet is one of the best ways to improve the chances of conceiving for women. Most women are worried about issues steaming from PCOS, which can cause a stop to your evolution cycle and make pregnancy impossible. But, recent studies showed that the women who were facing issues conceiving started conceiving when they chose a keto diet for themselves.

Keto can also help in different diseases, and most importantly, it helps improve your acne, which is normally a big hassle for women. It is also a cure for polycystic ovary syndrome and nervous system disorders.

Improve Neurological health:

Aging can put several neurological health risks, which include dementia and Alzheimer's disease. Research shows that it happens due to the increase of sugar level in the bloodstream, which causes these neurological diseases. Keeping these levels normal can help your brain work faster and improves your memory. Keto makes your neurological health better by reducing the intake of sugar in your diet. Weight gain is common for women when they are 50 or beyond, and this causes stress and neurological problem to some women. A Keto diet is the best way to improve your mental health and live life as you have dreamt of.

Combats fatigue:

Getting older and having a slower metabolism is a feeling which makes yourself so tired often, and you want to look younger and active at the same time. The best way to combat fatigue is to exercise and keep excess weight off. When you are on a Keto-friendly diet, you can snack as much as you can but definitely with the right foods. Your target can be burning your stubborn belly fats first because belly fats lead to visceral fats which squeezes internal organ and protect them from functioning in the right way.

Lowers your blood pressure:

Hypertension and increased blood pressure lead to significant risk factors for many diseases like kidney failure, stroke, and heart disease. Keto diet helps you lower your blood pressure and prevent you from these diseases. What do you need when you have a diet that is giving you a chance to live a longer life?

From a ketogenic diet, you get a chance to lose weight in days with a proper diet plan, which will allow your body to work in a better condition.

When you cut carbs, it becomes easier for you to lose weight in days. Every woman wants to look pretty and beautiful, and you also want to have a diet plan which is quick and easy for you to follow. Even though a low carb diet helps you lose weight in a short period but it has long-lasting benefits.

Improve the functioning of the immune system:

Keto diet is very advantageous for women because it provides women with a lot of health benefits. The concept of intermitted fasting in this diet is a blessing for women because it protects their immune system and reduces the risk of breast cancer. The other risks of women related diseases are also minimized when they are on a Keto diet.

Heal bone diseases like Arthritis:

Studies revealed that women over 50 who have arthritis were following a keto diet. Guess what? They healed from this diet, and their pain was gone away when they followed a specific diet plan and cut off carbs from their diet. Isn't it magical? Yes, you can also heal by following a keto diet. Some of you might be wondering if it would work on you, there is a great possibility that it will work on you.

Researchers have proved by several pieces of evidence that the keto diet is a perfect diet for women, and it is safe to start even if you are over 50. There is no harm to this diet if you are doing it right. You have to just make your mind and beat the aging stress from your mind. You would feel younger and healthier when you are on a Keto diet. It is a complete package which not only protects you from diseases but also gives you a chance to regain your energy and maintain ideal body weight. So, gear up, ladies! What are you waiting for?

Keto diet types

T he keto diet allows you to consume high-fat, low-carb foods. It also requires you to cut back on processed food items, sweets, starchy vegetables, and grains. If you're able to follow the diet well, you will be able to experience all the health benefits just like all the other individuals who have found success with this diet. The best thing about the keto diet is that there are a few types that you can choose from, including the following:

The Standard Ketogenic Diet, or SKD

The macronutrient ratio of this diet is 5–10 percent carbohydrates, 15–20 percent protein, and 75 percent fats. When you follow this diet, you need to plan all your snacks and meals around foods that are rich in fat. This is because you need to consume around 150 grams of fat each day so your body will start burning the fat for fuel. You also have to cut back on your carbohydrate intake, only eating 50 grams or less.

The Targeted Ketogenic Diet, or TKD

The macronutrient ratio of this diet is 10–15 percent carbohydrates, 20 percent protein, and 65–70 percent fat. This type of keto diet is very popular among active individuals, such as athletes. Unlike the standard keto diet, you're allowed to eat more carbohydrates right after or before working out.

The Cyclical Ketogenic Diet, or CKD

The macronutrient ratio of this diet is 5–10 percent carbohydrates, 15–20 percent protein, and 75 percent fat on "keto days." During "off days," the macronutrient ratio is 50 percent carbohydrates, 25 percent protein, and 25 percent fat. This type of keto diet allows you to cycle in and out of ketosis so that you can enjoy a balanced diet during your "off days."

The High-Protein Ketogenic Diet, or HPKD

The macronutrient ratio of this diet is 5–10 percent carbohydrates, 30 percent protein, and 60–65 percent fat. While following this type of keto diet, you should consume at least 120 grams of protein and 130 grams of fat each day. A lot of people prefer this diet because it allows them to consume less fat and more protein than the other types. However, following this diet might not allow you to achieve ketosis.

All about Ketosis

Ketosis refers to the natural state the body is in when it's almost completely fueled by fat. Ketosis occurs when you eat very little carbohydrates, moderate proteins, and a lot of fats. When your body runs out of glucose, it starts producing ketones, which, in turn, allows your body to achieve ketosis. There are different types of ketosis:

• *Fasting ketosis*—wherein your body reaches ketosis after you have fasted for a specific amount of time. Of course, the level of ketosis your body reaches will depend on how long you have been fasting.

• *Nutritional ketosis*—wherein your body reaches ketosis because of a modification in your diet. This type of ketosis includes *carbohydrate-restricted ketosis*, where you restrict the number of carbohydrates you consume. There's also *supplemental ketosis*, wherein you would take specific types of supplements for your body to achieve ketosis. And there's *alcoholic ketosis*, where you consume a lot of alcohol, which causes your body to become acidic because of the drastic increase of ketones.

• *Pathological ketosis*—also characterized by an acidic body environment. This type is the reason ketosis sometimes comes with a bad reputation.

After you have achieved ketosis, continue following the keto diet to maintain this body's natural state. This is important if you want to enjoy all the health benefits the keto diet has to offer.

The Keto Diet versus Other Low-Carb Diets

One common mistake a lot of people make is thinking that simply lowering their carbohydrate intake is already considered as following a keto diet. However, this isn't always the case because there are other types of low-carb diets out there, and they're not the same as the keto diet. A few of the low-carb diets might have some undesirable side effects on the body, unlike the keto diet.

If you just reduce the amounts of carbohydrates you eat or you avoid them altogether, you might experience some adverse side effects, such as fatigue, irritability, hormonal disruptions, weight gain, hunger pans, and more. Because some low-carb diets don't allow you to achieve ketosis, your body doesn't have an adequate source of fuel to function well. This is why if you plan to follow the keto diet to lose weight or to get all the health benefits, make sure to follow it properly.

What's the Difference between Low-Carb Diets and the Keto Diet?

Low-carb diets and the keto diet have been around for some time now, but as we've said, these two diets are different from each other. The effects they have on the body vary too; thus, you should know which type of diet you're following so you know exactly what types of foods to eat and avoid.

A low-carb diet involves eating minimal amounts of carbohydrates. The amount may differ from one diet to another, but the trouble with low-carb diets is that they don't consider the other types of macronutrients, such as proteins and fats. Conversely, the keto diet considers all the macronutrients in the equation, which gives your body an alternative source of fuel, which are the ketones. The great thing about the keto diet is that, unlike the other low-carb diets, you can measure your state of ketosis. This allows you to know if the diet is working.

How to Measure Ketones

Part of the keto diet is knowing how to measure your ketones. You need to know whether you have already reached ketosis or not to get the most out of this lifestyle choice. There are different ways to measure ketones:

• *Using a blood ketone meter.* This allows you to check your blood's ketone level precisely.

• *Using a breath test.* This measures your acetone levels.

• *Using a urine ketone test.* This can also be used for measuring ketones, but it's not as precise as the other methods and, therefore, might not be too reliable.

• *Using a test for blood glucose levels.* This measures your ketones by seeing how high or low your blood glucose levels are.

Ketogenic diet for women over 50

There is no uncertainty, ketogenic Diet has super advantages for ladies more than 50. Throughout the years, considers have discovered that limiting calories eases back maturing and builds life span - anyway the instrument of this impact has stayed tricky" Dr. Verdin said. , the paper's senior creator, coordinates the Center for HIV and Aging at Gladstone and is likewise a teacher at the University of California, San Francisco, with which Gladstone is associated. "Here, we find that βOHB - the body's significant wellspring of vitality during activity or fasting - obstructs a class of proteins that would somehow or another advance oxidative pressure, accordingly, shielding cells from maturing."

Oxidative pressure happens as cells use oxygen to deliver vitality, yet this action additionally discharges other conceivably harmful particles, known as free radicals. As cells age, they become less successful in clearing these free radicals - prompting cell harm, oxidative pressure and the impacts of maturing.

Insulin obstruction: Many senior residents in our general public are overweight and managing insulin-related conditions like diabetes. This is not kidding, as diabetes can prompt things like vision misfortune, kidney illness, and then some.

Bone wellbeing: Osteoporosis, in which decreased bone thickness makes bones delicate and fragile, is one of the most widely recognized conditions seen in more seasoned people. More calcium through day by day admission of milk items, as the USDA suggests, clearly isn't the appropriate response.

This is because the nations with the most noteworthy paces of osteoporosis will, in general, have the most noteworthy paces of dairy utilization. What's much better is to concentrate on a keto diet low in poisons, which meddle with retention, and is wealthy in all micronutrients as opposed to over-burden on a macronutrient (calcium).

Irritation: For some individuals, maturing incorporates more torment from wounds that occurred at a more youthful age or joint issues like joint inflammation.

Being in ketosis can help lessen the creation of substances considered cytokines that advance aggravation, which can help with these sorts of conditions.

Supplement lacks: Older grown-ups will, in general, have higher insufficiencies in significant supplements like:

Iron: lack can prompt mind mist and exhaustion

Vitamin B12: lack can prompt neurological conditions like dementia

Fats: lack can prompt issues with insight, skin, vision, and nutrient insufficiencies

Vitamin D: lack cause intellectual hindrance in more established grown-ups, increment the danger of coronary illness and even add to malignancy chance

The great wellsprings of creature protein on the ketogenic diet can without much of a stretch record for magnificent wellsprings of these significant supplements.

Controlling Blood Sugar: There is an association between poor glucose and mind related conditions like Alzheimer's illness, dementia, and Parkinson's disease. A few factors that may add to Alzheimer's sickness incorporate

An overabundance admission of starches, particularly from fructose—which is radically diminished in the ketogenic diet

An absence of dietary fats and cholesterol—which are rich and sound on the ketogenic diet

Oxidative pressure, which being in ketosis secures against

Utilizing a ketogenic diet to assist control with blooding sugar and improve nourishment may help improve insulin reaction as well as secure against memory issues that frequently occurred with age.

Significance of Keto for Aging

Keto nourishments convey a high measure of sustenance per calorie. This is significant because basal metabolic rate (the measure of calories required every day to endure) is less for seniors, however, they despite everything need an indistinguishable measure of supplements from more youthful individuals.

An individual age 50+ will have a lot harder time living on low-quality nourishments than a high schooler or 20-something whose body is flexible.

This makes it significantly increasingly urgent for seniors to eat nourishments that are wellbeing supporting and ailment battling. It can truly mean the contrast between getting a charge out of the brilliant years without limit or spending them in torment and distress.

In this manner, seniors need to eat a progressively ideal eating routine by keeping away from "void calories "from sugars or nourishments wealthy in enemies of supplements, for example, entire grains, and expanding their measure of supplement rich fats and proteins.

It is critical to monitor Ketogenic Diet by following your solid eating regimen with an exceptional clinical instrument at home without consulting your primary care physician each time.

Why for over 50

The ways that you take care of your body and the ways you stay active will dictate your quality of life and how good you will look. If you do not take care of your body, you might be fifty years old and look like you are sixty-five years old. But if you do good things for your body you might be sixty-five years old and look like you are fifty years old. Age really is just a number. And even if you haven't been active in a long time, or ever, it is never too late to start on some sort of activity plan to increase the quality of your life.

I call it an activity plan because no one really wants to exercise, right? So, let's think of this as an activity plan or a workout routine, both of those are positive statements that say you care about your body and you want to fight the effects of growing older with everything you've got.

Once a woman crosses that fifty-year mark, she begins losing one percent of her muscle each year. But muscle tone and fiber do not need to be lost with aging. With a proper workout, you can continue to build new muscle and maintain what you already have until you are in your nineties. And some of the exercises that you do for your muscles will help you build strong bones. This is especially important for women because losing the estrogen supplies in our bodies will cause us to lose bone mass faster than men do. This is when we are really at risk for developing osteoporosis.

And regular physical activity will help you to avoid developing that middle-age spread around the abdomen or to lose it if you already have it. Activity will help you to maintain a proper weight for your height and build which in turn will help you to avoid many, if not all, of the age-related, obesity-related diseases such as cardiovascular diseases and diabetes.

Physical activity comes in four main types. Each one should be done at least once or twice a week to ensure your body is getting the right mix of activity. The four main types of activity are:

Balance – Older people lose their sense of balance. It is easy for an older person to fall and break something, like a hip. When you engage in activities that help you to maintain your sense of balance will help reduce the risk that you might fall and suffer a permanent injury.

Stretching – As we age our muscles begin to lose their elasticity. This is part of why rolling out of bed in the morning gets more difficult as we get older. Stretching activities will help you to improve and maintain your level of flexibility which will help you to avoid injuries to your joints and muscles.

Cardiovascular/Aerobic – These are also called endurance activities because you should be able to maintain them for at least ten minutes at a time. This key here is to get your heart working faster and your breathing to be deeper. You should be working hard but still able to carry on a conversation. These activities will strengthen your heart and lungs which are, after all, very important muscles in your body.

Strength training – We are not talking about bodybuilding, but if you want to go for it. This will include working out with resistance bands or lifting weights. Either activity will help to build muscle.

While there are four separate categories of exercise that does not mean that you need to keep them strictly separated because many activities will encompass work in more than one area. You can lift light weights while doing balance activities. Walking and swimming will build muscle strength and cardiovascular health. Yoga will improve balance and assist with building muscle strength and stretching. The key is to engage in seventy-five minutes of vigorous activity each week, or fifteen minutes five days each week; or you can get one hundred fifty minutes of moderate activity in five thirty-minute sessions each week.

And make sure that you design a plan that fits you. Remember that it is perfectly fine to change your routine as your needs change. Maybe, in the beginning, you will work on balance three days each week because you really need help with that. But after a few weeks, your balance has improved enough so that you can devote one of those days to strength training. This is your routine made just for you so make it work for you. And don't forget to get your doctor's okay before beginning any type of activity routine. He will most likely give you his blessings but it is always good to ask. He can also provide you with information on activities that are good for you personally.

One thing to note here, especially if you have not been active in a while, is not to begin a vigorous level of activity the same day you begin the keto diet. During the time your body is getting used to the diet and going through ketosis, you will not feel like indulging in a lot of extra activity and your workout routine will be doomed to failure. This journey is all about making you the best you possibly can so don't sabotage yourself in the first few weeks. If you really want to start your activities on day one of your diet then I recommend walking or bicycling. Either of these activities can be started slowly, so a gentle walk or bike around the neighborhood after dinner is a perfect activity.

If you can get out and join a class at a local senior center, YMCA, community college, or church then do that. You will meet new people, some in your age group, and you can all work together to create your new bodies. But taking a class will not be the best choice for everyone. So we have included some basic exercises that can be done in the privacy of your home to get you started on the new lean you.

Stretching – Stretching activities are so important for older adults. These activities will also help you to improve your balance because you might find yourself standing or reaching in new and different ways.

Quad stretch – This is a simple exercise that can be done at home. Hold onto a chair or your partner for balance assistance if you need it. Then with the opposite hand lift the foot on that side behind you. Pull upward gently you can feel the beginning of a stretch in the front of your leg. As people get older, they may lean forward for balance and this muscle, the quad, can become shorter and less efficient over time. Hold this position steady for at least thirty seconds and repeat on the other side.

Hamstring stretch – This activity can be done on the sofa, the bed, or on the floor. Lay one leg in front of you and point your toes to the ceiling. Slowly fold your body over until you feel a stretching in the back of your leg and hold it for thirty seconds. NOTE: if you have recently had a hip replacement check with your doctor before doing this one.

Calf stretch – Place your hands on the wall and step back with one foot.

The back foot should be flat on the floor and the front knee should be slightly bent. Then lean forward toward the wall until you feel a stretch in your calf muscle. Hold it for thirty seconds and repeat on the other leg.

BALANCING – Balancing activities are so important for older adults to reduce the risk of falls. Tai Chi and Yoga are both excellent activities for assisting with better balance. You can find DVDs, routines online, or classes taught by certified instructors. Just remember to work with your body and your current level of ability and don't try to do an advanced routine if you have never mastered a beginner routine. You will just be setting yourself up for failure and we are here to succeed. And keep in mind that flexibility activities also help with the effects of arthritis. While you will want to explore the different types of yoga before making a decision on the one that is best for you, here is a yoga pose that anyone can do at home and helps to wake the whole body in the morning.

Mountain Pose – Stand straight with your feet together. Pull in your stomach muscles as tight as you can and let your shoulders relax. Keep your legs strong but do not lock your knees. Breathe deeply and regularly in and out for ten breaths.

Strength Training – This activity is especially important for you to ensure you keep your muscles strong and healthy for the next phase of your life. You can do many strength training activities without weights, or for an extra challenge add some light hand weights.

Punching – This will strengthen your arms and shoulders and get your blood moving at the same time. Stand straight with your feet apart slightly wider than your shoulders. Keep your stomach firm. Punch straight out with one fist and then the other for at least twenty repetitions.

Squat – This activity is great for strengthening the bottom and the thighs. This will help you to sit down – not fall down – and be able to rise from a seated position with ease and grace. Stand with your feet as far apart as your hips are wide to provide a stable stance. Push your bottom backward as you bend your knees. Your knees should never go out front further than your toes, and try to keep your weight over your heels. If you feel more secure this activity can be done in front of a chair in case you lose your balance and inadvertently sit down.

Bridge – Lie on your hind with your knees set and your feet at a distance as your hips. Keep your feet flat on the floor. Pull in your stomach and lift your hips to make a bridge of your back. Hold this pose for ten seconds and try to do at least ten.

Cardiovascular/Aerobic – The purpose here is to engage in some activity that gets your heart pumping faster and your lungs expanding further. Swimming, walking, running, cycling, aerobics classes, dancing – all of these are great activities for getting the circulation going again. Just remember to begin slowly and pay attention to your body. In other words, if something hurts, stop. But make sure it is really hurt. There is a difference between 'Wow I'm really out of shape because I haven't walked anywhere in a while' and 'My knee really hurts when I do that'. And any time you are ever in doubt seek medical attention.

Seated Activities –

The body will deteriorate if it is not used. Maybe you really want to engage in physical activities but you really can't stand up for long enough to do anything meaningful. You can sit down and do many activities that are designed to get you back into the routine of regular movement. Here are a few options for you:

Marching – sit tall in your chair with your feet flat on the floor and your legs bent at a ninety-degree angle. Lift one foot and then the other, as though you are marching in the chair. Raise the knee up in the air and keep the knee bent.

Shoulder Press – Sit tall in your chair. You can hold a set of light weights or simply make your hands into fists. If you do not own weights and do not want to buy any you can also use canned items or full water bottles. Raise your hands up into the air until your arms are straight and then lower them. Do these slowly so that your muscles will actually be doing the work.

Leg lifts – This activity will strengthen your quads, which is the muscle on the front of your leg. Strong quads are needed for walking upright. Sit tall in your chair with your knees bent at ninety degrees and your feet flat on the floor. Lift a foot up into the air and away from the chair slowly; let the muscle do the work. Hold the pose for five seconds and lower it. Repeat five times on each leg.

These are just a few of the activities that you can do to get yourself moving and help you in your weight loss and health goals. You are not too old to begin. You can find many routines on the internet so that you can use them alone in the privacy of your home.

Remember to preview a routine before you pay for anything in case you do not like it. And many routines are offered free of charge. So do a bit of research and don't stop with one activity. Try to make your routine as varied as possible so that you will not get bored and soon you will have that body you want along with a healthier you.

Keto side effects and how to solve them

In the 1st week of observing a Ketogenic diet and entering ketosis it is common to experience some side effects. You may suffer from headaches, tiredness, irritability, leg cramps , constipation and heart palpitations .

These side effects are usually relatively mild and temporary, and most of them can be avoided by consuming enough fluids and salt .

SIDE EFFECTS INCLUDES

Dizziness and headaches: this effect passes from the third day, it is the worst, the body has no energy and even if you get up quickly you can get dizzy.

Human brain needs glycogen (or ketone bodies) to be efficient from there this effect.

Bad breath: If there is an excess of ketone bodies in our bodies, it is advisable to drink plenty of water as these are released through breathing. Some people have a metallic taste in their mouth.

Urine with a very strong smell: ketone bodies are also eliminated in the urine so the smell of it becomes stronger.

Strong sweat: the smell is usually unpleasant because ketone bodies are also removed by sweat

Lack of appetite: In addition to the fact that it is much more expensive to digest than carbohydrates, protein and fat are very satisfying. Therefore, appetite is considerably reduced.

Nausea, vomiting, abdominal pain, respiratory distress and general decay

Loss of calcium: excess protein favors the loss of calcium by the kidney (which has previously been removed from the bones) and osteoporosis can be favored.

Possible arrhythmias: they may cause problems with the cardiac electrical conduction system and arrhythmias.

Loss of muscle: if it is a long time in ketosis, the fat is pulled first but when it is going down, the muscle begins to degrade to use its amino acids as fuel

The brain and its need for glycogen

Also note that he human brain has glucose as its food and therefore when it does not have glucose to feed it does it from ketone bodies. The problem with ketosis is that ketone bodies are acidic, and there are sources that claim that they can only be used by 50% by the brain and the rest must be supplied by glucose.

Keto 30 day keto meal plan for women over 50

Meal Plan	Breakfast	Lunch	Dinner	Snack
DAY-1	Berry Pancakes	Sweet Potato Casserole	Carolina-style Pork Barbecue	Soy Milk Yogurt
DAY-2	Quinoa Cakes	Chipotle Pomegranate Pulled Pork	Sweet and Sour Cabbage and Apples	Garlic Pumpkin Seeds
DAY-3	Artichoke Eggs	Keto Rack Of Lamb	Juicy and Peppery Tenderloin	Matcha Smoothie
DAY-4	Fruit Muffins	Spicy Butternut Squash Soup	Chipotle Pomegranate Pulled Pork	Jackfruit Coated Bites
DAY-5	Ginger French Toast	Healthy Avocado Beef Patties	Broccoli Cheese Soup	Pear Banana Spinach Smoothie Bowl
DAY-6	Avocado Egg Bake	Orange-maple Pork Roast	Butternut Squash and Carrot Soup	Coffee Cake

DAY-7	Aromatic Mushroom Bowl	Lovely Faux Mac and Cheese	Chicken Paprika With Spaghetti Squash	Cigar Borek
DAY-8	Quinoa Cakes	Hearty Beef & Sweet Potato Stew	Tantalizing Mushroom Gravy	Chickpea Slices
DAY-9	Morning Berry Salad	Caramelized Pork Chops and Onion	Ham Asparagus Soup	Matcha Smoothie
DAY-10	Vegetable Salad with Chickpeas	Zucchini Cream	Keto Rack Of Lamb With Port And Black Olive Sauce	Sofritas Tofu
DAY-11	Cherry Rice	Peanut Sesame Shirataki Noodles	Orange and Chili Garlic Sauce	Soy Milk Yogurt
DAY-12	Sausage Casserole	Thai Shrimp Soup	Easy Korean Beef	Choco Cake

DAY-13	Ginger French Toast	Cherry Chicken Lettuce Wraps	Healthy Avocado Beef Patties	Spirulina Green Smoothie Bowl
DAY-14	Grape Yogurt	Homemade Marinated Pork Roast	Chorizo Stuffed Summer Squash	Green Croquettes
DAY-15	Avocado Egg Bake	Chorizo Stuffed Summer Squash	Paprika Turkey Burgers	Tropical Green Paleo Smoothie
DAY-16	Morning Berry Salad	Provencal Lamb With Mediterranean Vegetables	Sweet Potato Casserole	Rice Porridge
DAY-17	Cherry Rice	Ravaging Beef Pot Roast	Broccoli Cheese Soup	Pear Banana Spinach Smoothie Bowl

DAY-18	Oven Baked Bacon	Sweet Potato Casserole	Curried Cheesy Cauliflower-squash Soup	Choco Cake
DAY-19	Dill Omelete	Sausage Mix	Lamb With Pecan-chipotle Sauce	Avocado Spinach Green Smoothie Bowl
DAY-20	Vegetable Salad with Chickpeas	Grilled Chicken with Lemon and Fennel	Cheesy Summer Squash Flatbreads	Sofritas Tofu
DAY-21	Sausage and Tomato Muffins	Chicken and Cabbage Platter	Sausage and Tomato Muffins	Pear Banana Spinach Smoothie Bowl
DAY-22	Salsa Eggs	Carolina-style Pork Barbecue	Sweet Potato Salad	Crunchy Oyster Mushrooms

DAY-23	Cheese Omelet	Chicken, Arugula & Butternut Squash Salad With Brussels Sprouts	Orange and Chili Garlic Sauce	Minty Alkaline Kiwi Green Smoothie
DAY-24	Cauliflower Hash Browns	Moist Cranberry Pork Roast	Grilled Chicken with Lemon and Fennel	Cigar Borek
DAY-25	Berry Pancakes	Peanut Sesame Shirataki Noodles	Rack Of Lamb With Figs	Polenta Fries
DAY-26	Cauliflower Hash Browns	Citrus-herb Pork Roast	Lemon-Garlic Chicken Thighs	Minty Alkaline Kiwi Green Smoothie
DAY-27	Oven Baked Bacon	Turkey and Brocolli soup	Lamb Rack With Cucumber Yogurt	Jackfruit Coated Bites

DAY-28	Artichoke Eggs	Easy Korean Beef	Pork 'n' Pepper Tortillas	Apple Crisp
DAY-29	Bean Casserole	Wrapped Asparagus	Chicken, Arugula & Butternut Squash Salad With Brussels Sprouts	Spirulina Green Smoothie Bowl
DAY-30	Poached Eggs Mytilene	Creamy Cauliflower Risotto	Rack Of Lamb With Figs	Green Croquettes

Breakfast recipes

1. Poached Eggs Mytilene

Preparation Time: 15 minutes

Cooking Time: 10 minutes

Servings: 1

Ingredients

Ground black pepper

½ juiced medium lemon

1 pinch salt

1 tbsp extra virgin olive oil

2 eggs

1 ½ tbsp white vinegar

1 ½ cups water

Directions

Get a small bowl and add in lemon juice and oil. Mix to combine.

Set your stove to medium high heat and in a small saucepan put water and vinegar to boil. Turn the heat down to medium low, and now it's time to cook your eggs. Break them carefully into the boiling water. You want to be careful not to disturb the yolk. Let the eggs cook for 3 minutes. You are shooting for firm whites and a mildly cooked yolk.

Take out the eggs using a slotted spoon and put into a seperate serving bowl.

Pour the lemon-oil onto the eggs and beat with a fork. Mix properly and add some salt and pepper.

This will fit well in a bowl of avocado toast with tomato. Place it over your homemade salad.

Nutrition:

Calories:275;

Carbohydrates: 3.9g;

Protein: 5.6g; Fat: 23.6g;

Sugar: 0.3g; Sodium: 307mg;

Fiber: 1.9g

2. Cauliflower Hash Browns

Preparation Time: 15 minutes

Cooking Time: 25 minutes

Servings: 1

Ingredients

Cooking spray

3 cups grated cauliflower

1 pinch cayenne pepper

1 cup cheddar cheese, shredded

Pinch ground black pepper

1 large egg

½ tsp salt

¼ cup real bacon bits

1 tbsp chives, chopped

Directions: *Ensure that you heat your oven to 400 degrees F before you start cooking. To proceed, you'll need a bowl that is microwave-safe. Set the microwave to high and, after adding your cauliflower to the bowl, cook for 2 minutes. Afterwards, take the bowl out and set it aside for 5 minutes.*

Squeeze out as much fluid as you can from the cauliflower with the help of a dish towel.

Place the cauliflower, cayenne pepper, cheddar cheese, black pepper, egg, salt, bacon, and chives into a mixing bowl. Mix properly to combine the ingredients.

Prepare a baking sheet by oiling it with cooking spray. Separate the cauliflower into 6 parts. Press down with your hands and mold them into oval shapes.

It's time to bake. Toss it in the oven and let it cook for 15 minutes. Set the broiler to low and cook the hash brown to a crispy texture. This should take 5 minutes.

Set it aside for an additional 5 minutes before you serve.

Nutrition: Calories: 118

Carbohydrates: 3g;

Protein: 8.8g; Fat: 8.2g; Sugar: 54g; Sodium: 484mg;

Fiber: 2.3g

3. Fluffy Scrambled Eggs

Preparation Time: 5 minutes

Cooking Time: 5 minutes

Servings: 2

Ingredients

Pinch salt

4 eggs - ¼ cup milk

Directions

Get a mixing bowl that can survive in a microwave. Crack open the eggs into the bowl, and add your salt and milk. Mix well to combine.

Turn the microwave to high and place in the bowl. After about 30 seconds, take the bowl out and beat the eggs. Pop back into the microwave and cook for 30 seconds. Repeat this pattern for a total of 2 ½ minutes.

Nutrition: Calories:141; Carbohydrates: 2.1g; Protein: 12.1g; Fat: 9.3g; Sugar: 2g; Sodium: 281mg; Fiber: 2.4g

4. Oven Baked Bacon

Preparation Time: 5 minutes

Cooking Time: 30 minutes

Servings: 6

Ingredients

16 oz pack bacon

Directions

Preheat the oven to 350 degrees F. Use parchment paper to line a baking sheet.

Arrange the slices of bacon on the baking sheet. Next, bake them in your oven for 20 minutes. Take out the baking sheet to turn the slices. Place the baking sheet back in the oven to cook the other side. After another 20 minutes, Your bacon should be ready. Line a plate with clean paper towels, and drain the bacon with them.

Nutrition: Calories:134; Carbohydrates: 0.9g; Protein: 5.6g; Fat: 10.4g; Sugar: 1g; Sodium: 547mg; Fiber: 1.3g

5. Avocado Egg Bake

Preparation Time: 5 minutes

Cooking Time: 15 minutes

Servings: 1

Ingredients

1 tbsp fresh parsley, chopped

1 avocado, cut in half and the pits removed

Salt to your preferred taste

Ground black pepper to your preferred taste

2 eggs

¼ cup cheddar cheese shredded

Directions

Preheat the oven to 425 degrees F.

The next thing to do is scoop some avocado from the pitted area. Place both halves of the avocado on a baking sheet and break an egg onto each avocado.

Let it bake in the oven for about 20 minutes. Only stop bakin when you are sure the eggs are cooked. Add salt and pepper to season the avocado egg, and garnish with cheddar cheese and parsley.

Nutrition:

Calories:605;

Carbohydrates: 18.6g;

Protein: 25.6g;

Fat: 50.9g;

Sugar: 3.8g;

Sodium: 525mg;

Fiber: 6.6g

6. Salsa Eggs

Preparation Time: 10 minutes

Cooking Time: 10 minutes

Servings: 4

Ingredients

2 tomatoes, chopped

1 chili pepper, chopped

2 cucumbers, chopped

1 red onion, chopped

2 tablespoons parsley, chopped

1 tablespoon olive oil

1 tablespoon lemon juice

4 eggs

1 cup water, for cooking eggs

Directions

Put eggs in the water and boil them for 7 minutes. Cool the cooked eggs in the cold water and peel. After this, make salsa salad: mix up tomatoes, chili pepper, cucumbers, red onion, parsley, olive oil, and lemon juice.

Cut the eggs into the halves and sprinkle generously with cooked salsa salad.

Nutrition:

Calories:140;

Carbohydrates: 8.3g;

Protein: 11.1g;

Fat: 2.2g;

Sugar: 2.7g;

Sodium: 484mg;

Fiber: 164g

7. Fruit Scones

Preparation Time: 10 minutes

Cooking Time: 12 minutes

Servings: 8

Ingredients: ¼ cup chia seeds

2 cups whole-grain wheat flour

½ teaspoon baking powder

¼ cup cranberries, dried

¼ cup apricots, chopped

¼ cup almonds, chopped

1 tablespoon liquid honey

1 egg, whisked

Directions

In the bowl mix up all the ingredients and knead the dough.

Cut the dough into 16 pieces (scones). Bake them at 350 degrees F for 12 minutes in the lined with baking paper tray. Cool the scones well.

Nutrition: Calories:156;

Carbohydrates: 3.6g;

Protein: 27.1g; Fat: 2.9g;

Sugar: 0.2g; Sodium: 216mg;

Fiber: 220g

8. Cheese Omelet

Preparation Time: 10 minutes

Cooking Time: 10 minutes

Servings: 4

Ingredients

1 tablespoon olive oil

½ teaspoon ground black pepper

1 cup baby spinach, chopped

3 eggs, beaten

2 oz low-fat Low-fat feta cheese, crumbled

1 tablespoons cilantro, chopped

Directions: Heat up a pan with the oil over the medium-high heat, add spinach and saute for 3 minutes. Then add all remaining ingredients and stir gently. Close the lid and cook an omelet for 7 minutes on low heat or until it is solid.

Nutrition: Calories:117;

Carbohydrates: 9.8g;

Protein: 1.3g; Fat: 0.3g;

Sugar: 1.5g; Sodium: 211mg;

Fiber: 135g

9. Berry Pancakes

Preparation Time: 10 minutes

Cooking Time: 10 minutes

Servings: 8

Ingredients: 2 eggs, whisked

4 tablespoons almond milk

1 cup low-fat yogurt

3 tablespoons margarine, melted

½ teaspoon vanilla extract

1 cup almond flour

1 cup strawberries

Directions: Pour the margarine in the skillet.

Mix up all remaining ingredients and blend with the help of the mixer.

Then pour the dough in the hot skillet in the shape of the pancakes and cook for 1.5 minutes from each side.

Nutrition: Calories:80;

Carbohydrates: 6.2g;

Protein: 3.3g; Fat: 6.2g;

Sugar: 0.3g; Sodium 0mg;

Fiber: 29g

10. Strawberry Sandwich

Preparation Time: 5 minutes

Cooking Time: 0 minutes

Servings: 4

Ingredients

4 tablespoons low-fat yogurt

4 strawberries, sliced

4 whole-wheat bread slices

Directions

Spread the bread with yogurt and then top with sliced strawberries.

Nutrition:

Calories:84;

Carbohydrates: 1.2g;

Protein: 4.6g;

Fat: 1.2g;

Sugar: 4g;

Sodium: 124mg;

Fiber: 2.1g

11. Ginger French Toast

Preparation Time: 5 minutes

Cooking Time: 10 minutes

Servings: 2

Ingredients

4 whole-wheat bread slices

½ cup low-fat milk

2 eggs, whisked

1 teaspoon ground ginger

Cooking spray

Directions

Spray the skillet with cooking spray.

In the mixing bowl mix up milk and eggs.

Then add ginger and dip the bread in the liquid.

Roast the bread in the preheated skillet for 2 minutes from each side.

Nutrition: Calories:229;

Carbohydrates: 8g;

Protein: 29.4g; Fat: 8g;

Sugar: 2g;

Sodium: 388mg; Fiber: 4g

12. Fruit Muffins

Preparation Time: 10 minutes

Cooking Time: 35 minutes

Servings: 6

Ingredients 1 cup apple, grated

1 cup quinoa 2 cups oatmeal

½ cup of coconut milk

1 tablespoon liquid honey

1 teaspoon vanilla extract

1 tablespoon olive oil

1 cup of water

1 teaspoon ground nutmeg

Directions

Mix up water and quinoa and the mixture for 15 minutes, fluff with a fork and transfer to a bowl.Add all remaining ingredients and mix up well. Transfer the batter in the muffin molds and bake them at 375F for 20 minutes.

Nutrition: Calories:308;

Carbohydrates: 46g;

Protein: 8.2g; Fat:10 .8g;

Sugar: 3g; Sodium: 355mg;

Fiber: 6.2g

13. Omelet with Peppers

Preparation Time: 10 minutes

Cooking Time: 15 minutes

Servings: 4

Ingredients

4 eggs, beaten

1 tablespoon margarine

1 cup bell peppers, chopped

2 oz scallions, chopped

Directions

Toss the margarine in the skillet and melt it.

In the mixing bowl mix up eggs and bell peppers. Add scallions. Pour the egg mixture in the hot skillet and roast the omelet for 12 minutes.

Nutrition:

Calories:102;

Carbohydrates: 7.3g;

Protein: 6.1g;

Fat: 10 .8g;

Sugar: 3g;

Sodium: 98mg;

Fiber: 0.8g

14. Quinoa Hashes

Preparation Time: 10 minutes

Cooking Time: 25inutes

Servings: 2

Ingredients

3 oz quinoa

6 oz water

2 potatoes, grated

1 egg, beaten

1 tablespoon avocado oil

1 teaspoon chives, chopped

Directions

Cook quinoa in water for 15 minutes.

Heat up avocado oil in the skillet.

Then mix up all remaining ingredients in the bowl. Add quinoa and mix up well.

Add quinoa hash browns, cook for 5 minutes on each side.

Nutrition: Calories:344;

Carbohydrates: 5.9g;

Protein: 12.5.g; Fat: 5.9g;

Sugar: 0.2g; Sodium: 388mg;

Fiber: 3.4g

15. Artichoke Eggs

Preparation Time: 5 minutes

Cooking Time: 20 minutes

Servings: 4

Ingredients

5 eggs, beaten

2 oz low-fat feta, chopped

1 yellow onion, chopped

1 tablespoon canola oil

1 tablespoon cilantro, chopped

1 cup artichoke hearts, canned, chopped

Directions

Grease 4 ramekins with the oil.

Mix up all remaining ingredients and divide the mixture between prepared ramekins.

Bake the meal at 380F for 20 minutes.

Nutrition:

Calories:177;

Carbohydrates: 7.4g;

Protein: 10.6g;

Fat: 12.2g; Sugar: 1g;

Sodium: 259mg; Fiber: 2g

16. Quinoa Cakes

Preparation Time: 10 minutes

Cooking Time: 25 minutes

Servings: 4

Ingredients

7 oz quinoa

1 cup cauliflower, shredded

1 cup of water

½ cup vegan parmesan, grated

1 egg, beaten

1 tablespoon olive oil

½ teaspoon ground black pepper

 Directions

Mix up the quinoa with the cauliflower, water, and ground black pepper, stir, bring to a simmer over medium heat and cook for 15 minutes/

Cool the mixture and add parmesan and the eggs, stir well, shape medium cakes out of this mix.

Heat up a pan with the oil over medium-high heat, add the quinoa cakes. Cook them for 4-5 minutes per side.

Nutrition:

Calories:280;

Carbohydrates: 6.8g;

Protein: 25.4g;

Fat: 7.6g;

Sugar: 1.2g;

Sodium: 222mg;

Fiber: 1g

17. Bean Casserole

Preparation Time: 10 minutes

Cooking Time: 30 minutes

Servings: 8

Ingredients

5 eggs, beaten

½ cup bell pepper, chopped

1 cup red kidney beans, cooked

½ cup white onions, chopped

1 cup low-fat mozzarella cheese, shredded

Directions

Spread the beans over the casserole mold. Add onions and bell pepper.

Add the eggs mixed with the cheese.

Bake the casserole 380 F for 30 minutes.

Nutrition:

Calories:142;

Carbohydrates: 16g;

Protein: 23.8g;

Fat: 3g;

Sugar: 0.2g;

Sodium: 162mg;

Fiber: 2.3g

18. Grape Yogurt

Preparation Time: 10 minutes

Cooking Time: 0 minutes

Servings: 3

Ingredients

1 ½ cup low-fat yogurt

½ cup grapes, chopped

1 oz walnuts, chopped

Directions

Mix up all ingredients together and transfer them in the serving glasses.

Nutrition:

Calories:156;

Carbohydrates: 12.2g;

Protein: 9.4g;

Fat: 8g;

Sugar: 5.6g;

Sodium: 88mg;

Fiber: 0.7g

19. Vegetables with Hash Browns

Preparation Time: 10 minutes

Cooking Time: 20 minutes

Servings: 5

Ingredients

1 tablespoon canola oil

4 eggs, beaten

7 oz hash browns

4 oz low-fat cheese, shredded

1 small onion, diced

½ teaspoon chili flakes

1 green bell pepper, chopped

1 carrot, shredded

1 tablespoon parsley, chopped

Directions

Heat up oil in the pan and add hash browns and onion. Cook the mixture for 5 minutes.

Add the bell peppers and the carrots, toss and cook for 5 minutes more.

Then add eggs, black pepper, and the cheese, stir and cook for another 10 minutes.

Add the parsley, stir and cook for 10 seconds more.

Nutrition:

Calories:290;

Carbohydrates: 18.9g;

Protein: 11.8g;

Fat: 16g;

Sugar: 7g;

Sodium: 336mg;

Fiber: 2g

20. Berry Quinoa

Preparation Time: 10 minutes

Cooking Time: 20 minutes

Servings: 4

Ingredients

1 cup white quinoa

2 cups of water

2 tablespoons lemon juice

2 tablespoon liquid honey

1 teaspoon dried mint

1 cup blackberries

1 cup strawberries, sliced

1 cup mango, chopped

Directions

Cook quinoa in water for 20 minutes.

Then add blackberries, strawberries, and mango and toss.

Add lemon juice, mint, and honey. Stir well.

Nutrition: Calories:128;

Carbohydrates: 8g;

Protein: 28.4g; Fat: 1.5g;

Sugar: 1g; Sodium: 201mg;

Fiber: 0.5g

21. Scallions Risotto

Preparation Time: 10 minutes

Cooking Time: 20 minutes

Servings: 4

Ingredients

4 slices bacon, low-sodium, chopped

1 tablespoon olive oil

1 cup white rice, cooked

2 tablespoons low-fat mozzarella, grated

2 tablespoons scallions, chopped

½ teaspoon white pepper

Directions

Heat up a pan with the oil over medium-high heat, add the bacon and cook it for 5 minutes. Add all remaining ingredients and cook them for 15 minutes over medium heat.

Nutrition: Calories:241; Carbohydrates: 37.9g; Protein: 7.4g; Fat: 6.4g; Sugar: 3g; Sodium: 91mg; Fiber: 3g

22. Vegetable Salad with Chickpeas

Preparation Time: 10 minutes

Cooking Time: 0 minutes

Servings: 4

Ingredients

1 tablespoon cilantro, chopped

1 tablespoon scallions, chopped

1 cups radishes, chopped

1 apple, cored, peeled and cubed

1 teaspoon coriander, ground

3 tablespoons olive oil

2 cups chickpeas, cooked

1 chili pepper, chopped

1 tablespoon lemon juice

Directions

Mix up all ingredients in the salad bowl.

Shake the salad well before serving.

Nutrition: Calories:490; Carbohydrates: 6.5g; Protein: 29.4g; Fat: 6g; Sugar: 2.2g; Sodium: 254mg; Fiber: 1.7g

23. Cherry Rice

Preparation Time: 10 minutes

Cooking Time: 25 minutes

Servings: 4

Ingredients

1 cup low-fat milk

1 cup white rice

½ teaspoon vanilla extract

¼ cup cherries, pitted and halved

Directions

Put the milk in a pot and add rice.

Simmer the mixture for 25 minutes stirring often.

Add all remaining ingredients and mix up well.

Nutrition:

Calories:201;

Carbohydrates: 5.5g;

Protein: 5.4g;

Fat: 7g;

Sugar: 0.2g;

Sodium: 258mg;

Fiber: 0.4g

24. Morning Berry Salad

Preparation Time: 10 minutes

Cooking Time: 0 minutes

Servings: 4

Ingredients

4 cups salad greens, chopped

4 cups blackberries

3 cups orange, chopped

For the vinaigrette:

1 cup olive oil

2 teaspoons shallot, minced

½ teaspoon ground paprika

Directions

Blend together all the ingredients for the vinaigrette.

Then mix up all remaining ingredients in the salad bowl.

Add the vinaigrette and shake it well.

Nutrition:

Calories:396;

Carbohydrates: 24.5g;

Protein: 4.2g;

Fat: 34.2g;

Sugar: 2.2g;

Sodium: 308mg; Fiber: 0.3g

25. Sausage Casserole

Preparation Time: 10 minutes

Cooking Time: 35 minutes

Servings: 4

Ingredients

2 eggs, beaten

1 onion, chopped

1 chili pepper, chopped

1 tablespoon olive oil

1 cup ground sausages

1 teaspoon chili flakes

Directions

Mix up olive oil, onion, and ground sausages in the pan.

Add all remaining ingredients and mix up the mixture well. Roast the mixture for 5 minutes.

Then transfer it in the oven and bake at 370F for 25 minutes.

Nutrition: Calories:73;

Carbohydrates: 5.5g;

Protein: 8.4g; Fat: 4.6g;

Sugar: 0.2g; Sodium: 584mg;

Fiber: 4.6g

26. Dill Omelet

Preparation Time: 10 minutes

Cooking Time: 6 minutes

Servings: 4

Ingredients

2 tablespoons low-fat milk

¼ teaspoon white pepper

6 eggs, beaten

2 tablespoons dill, chopped

1 tablespoon avocado oil

Directions

Heat up avocado oil in the skillet.

In a bowl, mix up all ingredients.

Pour the egg mixture in the hot oil and cook the omelet for 6 minutes.

Nutrition:

Calories:90;

Carbohydrates: 1.4g;

Protein: 9g;

Fat: 4.8g;

Sugar: 0.2g;

Sodium: 408mg; Fiber: 0.4g

27. Aromatic Mushroom Bowl

Preparation Time: 10 minutes

Cooking Time: 30 minutes

Servings: 4

Ingredients

1 white onion, chopped

1 cup quinoa

1 teaspoon minced garlic

2 tablespoons olive oil

1 cup of water

1 tablespoon cilantro, chopped

½ pound white mushroom, sliced

Directions

Heat up a pan with the oil over medium heat, add the onion, garlic, and mushrooms, stir and cook for 5-6 minutes.

Boil quinoa with water in the pan for 15 minutes.

Then transfer the quinoa and cooked mushroom mixture in the serving bowls. Top the meal with cilantro.

Nutrition:

Calories:347;

Carbohydrates: 22g;

Protein: 34g;

Fat: 9.8g;

Sugar: 3.1g;

Sodium: 332mg;

Fiber: 0.5g

Appetizer Recipes

28. Dill Cucumber Cups

Preparation Time: 10 minutes

Cooking Time: 0 minutes

Servings: 1

Ingredients:

2 eggs, hard boiled, peeled and sliced

1 cucumber, cut into medium slices

1 tablespoon fresh dill, chopped

¼ teaspoon sweet paprika

Salt and ground black pepper, to taste

Directions:

Arrange the cucumber slices on a plate, add the egg slices on top, add the rest of the ingredients as well and serve as an appetizer.

Nutrition: Calories:170; Carbohydrates: 2g; Protein: 14g; Fat: 5g; Sugar: 2.2g; Sodium: 254mg; Fiber: 0g

29. Turkey Wraps

Preparation Time: 10 minutes

Cooking Time: 0 minutes

Servings: 2

Ingredients:

6 chives, 2 of them chopped

4 ounces turkey breast, cooked and cut into 8 pieces

1 peach, cut into 8 wedges

Directions:

Roll 2 peach wedges and some of the minced chives in 2 slices of turkey.

Wrap this roll in 1 chive, repeat with the remaining ingredients and serve as an appetizer.

Nutrition: Calories:180; Carbohydrates: 12g; Protein: 29.4g; Fat: 2g; Sugar: 3.1g; Sodium: 128mg; Fiber: 3.3g

30. Chips and Mango Salsa

Preparation Time: 10 minutes

Cooking Time: 6 minutes

Servings: 4

Ingredients:

4 green plantains, peeled and thinly sliced

4 cups coconut oil, melted

Salt

For the mango salsa:

1 avocado, pitted, peeled, and cubed

2 cups mango, cubed

¼ cup fresh cilantro, chopped

½ cup onion, chopped

2 tablespoons olive oil

Salt and ground black pepper, to taste

Juice of 1 lime

A pinch of red pepper flakes

Directions:

Heat a pan with the coconut oil over medium-high heat, add the plantain chips, cook them for about 6 minutes, drain excess grease on paper towels and divide them into bowls.

In a bowl, mix the mango with the remaining ingredients, toss and serve the chips with this.

Nutrition:

Calories:200;

Carbohydrates: 8g;

Protein: 14g;

Fat: 3g;

Sugar: 2.2g;

Sodium: 432mg;

Fiber: 0g

31. Kale Chips

Preparation Time: 10 minutes

Cooking Time: 1 hour 30 minutes

Servings: 10

Ingredients:

1 bunch kale, trimmed and leaves separated

Salt and ground black pepper, to taste

3 tablespoons olive oil

Juice of 1 lemon

⅔ cup jarred roasted peppers

¼ teaspoon chili powder

½ teaspoon garlic powder

Directions:

In a food processor, mix the roasted pepper with the oil, salt, pepper, lemon juice, chili powder and garlic powder and pulse really well.

On a baking sheet, combine the kale with the pepper mix, toss, bake at 400 degrees F for 1 hour and 30 minutes tossing them halfway and serve cold.

Nutrition:

Calories:126;

Carbohydrates: 4g;

Protein: 12g;

Fat: 6g;

Sugar: 4g;

Sodium: 365mg;

Fiber: 1g

32. Green Beans Bowls

Preparation Time: 10 minutes

Cooking Time: 8hours

Servings: 8

Ingredients:

⅓ cup olive oil

5 pounds green beans, trimmed

A pinch of salt and black pepper

1 teaspoon garlic powder

1 teaspoon onion powder

Directions:

In a bowl, mix the beans with salt, pepper and the other ingredients, toss, put them in a dehydrator and dry them at 135 degrees F for 8 hours.

Serve them as a snack.

Nutrition:

Calories:90;

Carbohydrates: 6g;

Protein: 10g;

Fat: 3g;

Sugar: 0g;

Sodium: 345mg;

Fiber: 0g

33. Dates Bowl

Preparation Time: 10 minutes

Cooking Time: 0 minutes

Servings: 4

Ingredients:

2 medjool dates, cut on one side

5 pistachios, raw and chopped

1 teaspoon coconut, shredded

Directions:

Stuff each date with the pistachios and coconut, transfer to a bowl and serve.

Nutrition:

Calories:60;

Carbohydrates: 0.2g;

Protein: 4g;

Fat: 2g;

Sugar: 0g;

Sodium: 254mg;

Fiber: 0g

34. Cocoa Balls

Preparation Time: 15 hours

Cooking Time: 0 minutes

Servings: 12

Ingredients:

3 cups brewed coffee, cold

1 cup raw almonds

2 tablespoons cocoa powder

10 dates

2 teaspoons instant coffee

Directions:

In a bowl, mix the almonds with the coffee, set aside for about 1 hour, drain the almonds, transfer them to a food processor, add the coffee and the other ingredients, pulse, shape medium balls out of this, divide into bowls and serve as a snack.

Nutrition: Calories:50;

Carbohydrates: 8g; Protein: 1g;

Fat: 2g; Sugar: 0g;

Sodium: 107mg;

Fiber: 1g

35. Fruit and Nut Snack

Preparation Time: 10 minutes

Cooking Time: 12 minutes

Servings: 8

Ingredients:

1 cup dried fruits

1 cup dates, pitted and dried

1 cup mixed nuts

Directions:

Arrange nuts on a lined baking sheet and roast in the oven at 350°F for 12 minutes.

In a bowl, mix the nuts with the rest of the ingredients, toss, divide into bowls and serve as a snack.

Nutrition:

Calories:200;

Carbohydrates: 41g;

Protein: 4g;

Fat: 7g;

Sugar: 0.3g;

Sodium: 458mg;

Fiber: 0g

36. Garlic Chinese Chips

Preparation Time: 10 minutes

Cooking Time: 15 minutes

Servings: 6

Ingredients: **12 nori sheets**

1 tablespoon olive oil

¼ cup water

Salt and ground black pepper, to taste

3 garlic cloves, peeled and minced

Directions: Place 6 nori sheets on a lined baking sheet, brush with water, top them with the other 6 sheets, cut them all into thin strips, drizzle the oil, season with salt, pepper and the garlic and cook at 300 degrees F for 15 minutes.

Divide into bowls and serve cold.

Nutrition: Calories:42;

Carbohydrates: 3g;

Protein: 2.4g; Fat: 5g;

Sugar: 0g; Sodium: 254mg;

Fiber: 0g

37. Spinach Chips

Preparation Time: 10 minutes

Cooking Time: 10 minutes

Servings: 3

Ingredients:

2 cups baby spinach, washed

Salt and ground black pepper, to taste

2 teaspoons garlic, minced

½ tablespoon olive oil

Directions:

On a lined baking sheet, combine the spinach with the rest of the ingredients, toss, spread them well, place in the oven and bake at 400° F for 10 minutes.

Serve cold as a snack.

Nutrition:

Calories:75;

Carbohydrates: 2.5g;

Protein: 2g;

Fat: 4g;

Sugar: 0.3g;

Sodium: 154mg;

Fiber: 0g

38. Chicken Dip

Servings: 4

Cooking Time: 50 minutes

Preparation Time: 10 minutes

Ingredients:

1 pound chicken meat, cooked and shredded

½ cup mayonnaise

3 tablespoons cilantro, chopped

1 onion, peeled and chopped

For the sauce:

15 ounces tomato sauce

4 teaspoons mustard

¼ cup apple cider vinegar

2 teaspoons chili powder

Salt and ground black pepper, to taste

2 teaspoons onion powder

Directions:

Heat a small pot over medium heat, add the tomato sauce, vinegar, mustard, chili powder, onion powder, salt, and pepper, stir, bring to a boil, cook for 20 minutes, take off the heat and transfer to a baking dish.

Add the chicken and the rest of the ingredients, bake at 350 degrees F for 20 minutes, divide into small bowls and serve as a party dip.

Nutrition:

Calories:130;

Carbohydrates: 6g;

Protein: 9g;

Fat: 2g;

Sugar: 2.1g;

Sodium: 554mg;

Fiber: 0g

39. Zucchini Dip

Preparation Time: 10 minutes

Cooking Time: 20 minutes

Servings: 4

Ingredients:

2 zucchinis, chopped

Salt and ground black pepper, to taste

1 tablespoon olive oil

4 garlic cloves, peeled and chopped

½ cup sesame seeds paste

2 tablespoons lemon juice

4 ounces roasted bell peppers, chopped

Directions:

Arrange the zucchini on a baking sheet, drizzle the oil, add the salt and pepper, toss to coat, bake in the oven at 400°F for 20 minutes, cool them down, and transfer to a food processor. Add the rest of the ingredients, pulse, divide into small bowls and serve as a party dip.

Nutrition:

Calories:140;

Carbohydrates: 6g;

Protein: 8g;

Fat: 4g;

Sugar: 0g;

Sodium: 254mg;

Fiber: 0g

40. Chicken Bites and Mint Dip

Preparation Time: 10 minutes

Cooking Time: 20 minutes

Servings: 6

Ingredients:

2 chicken breast, cut into thin strips

1 cup coconut flour

½ cup coconut, shredded

1 teaspoon dry mustard

1 teaspoon garlic powder

1 teaspoon sweet paprika

2 tablespoons sesame seeds

Salt and ground black pepper, to taste

3 tablespoons olive oil

2 eggs

For the dip:

Zest and juice from 1 lemon

4 mint sprigs, chopped

1 small garlic clove, minced

Salt and ground black pepper, to taste

Directions:

In a bowl, whisk the eggs well.

In another bowl, whisk the flour with the coconut and the other ingredients except the oil and the ones for the dip and whisk.

Dip the chicken in the egg and then in almond mix, arrange them on a lined baking sheet, drizzle the olive oil over them, and bake in the oven at 400°F for 15 minutes.

In a bowl, mix the lemon juice with the rest of the ingredients, whisk and serve the chicken bites with this.

Nutrition:

Calories:300;

Carbohydrates: 11g;

Protein: 25g;

Fat: 8g;

Sugar: 0g;

Sodium: 508mg;

Fiber: 3g

41. Eggplant Platter

Preparation Time: 10 minutes

Cooking Time: 25 minutes

Servings: 6

Ingredients:

2 eggplants, sliced

½ cup coconut flour

3 egg whites, whisked

2 teaspoons olive oil

¼ teaspoon sweet paprika

Salt and ground black pepper, to taste

16 ounces chorizo, cooked and diced

3 garlic cloves, peeled and minced

1 onion, peeled and chopped

1 tomato, cored and chopped

¼ cup fresh basil, chopped

Directions:

In a bowl, mix flour with the salt, pepper, and paprika.

Put the egg white in a second bowl. Dip eggplant slices in the egg white, then in the flour mixture, place them on a lined baking sheet, drizzle the oil over them, cook at 350°F for 25 minutes and arrange them on a platter. In another bowl, mix the rest of the ingredients, toss, spread this over the eggplant and serve.

Nutrition:

Calories:160;

Carbohydrates: 6g;

Protein: 12g;

Fat: 3g;

Sugar: 0g;

Sodium: 124mg;

Fiber: 1g

42. Potato Bites

Preparation Time: 10 minutes

Cooking Time: 20 minutes

Servings: 3

Ingredients:

1 potato, sliced

2 bacon slices, cooked and crumbled

1 small avocado, pitted and cubed

A drizzle of olive oil

4 eggs, hard boiled, peeled and sliced

Directions:

Arrange the potato slices on a lined baking sheet, drizzle the oil, bake in the oven at 350°F for 20 minutes, arrange them on a platter, top each with the rest of the ingredients and serve as an appetizer.

Nutrition:

Calories:140;

Carbohydrates: 8g;

Protein: 9g;

Fat: 4g;

Sugar: 0g;

Sodium: 408mg;

Fiber: 1.7g

43. Egg Cups

Preparation Time: 10 minutes

Cooking Time: 0 minutes

Servings: 12

Ingredients: 1teaspoon mustard

6 eggs, hard boiled, peeled and cut into halves lengthwise and yolks separated

Salt and ground black pepper, to taste - ¼ cup homemade mayonnaise - 1 teaspoon white vinegar - 1 avocado, pitted, peeled, and chopped

3.5 ounces smoked salmon, flaked -A handful fresh cilantro, chopped

Directions: In a bowl, mix the egg yolks with mustard and the other ingredients except the egg halves, stir, stuff the egg halves with this and serve as an appetizer.

Nutrition: Calories:89; Protein: 12g; Carbohydrates: 5g; Fat: 4g; Sugar: 0.4g; Sodium: 120mg; Fiber: 0g

44. Mushroom Bites

Preparation Time: 10 minutes

Cooking Time: 25 minutes

Servings: 12

Ingredients:

1 pound pork sausage, chopped

1 tablespoon olive oil

1 red bell pepper, seeded and chopped

1 onion, peeled and chopped

2 pounds button mushrooms caps

3 garlic cloves, peeled and minced

2 cups spinach, chopped

Salt and ground black pepper, to taste

¼ cup fresh cilantro, chopped

Directions:

Heat a pan with the oil over medium heat, add the bell pepper and onion, stir, and cook for 3 minutes. Add the garlic and the rest of the ingredients except the mushroom caps, cook for 2 more minutes and stuff each mushroom with this mixture.

Arrange them on a lined baking sheet, bake them in the oven at 350°F for 20 minutes, arrange on a platter and serve as an appetizer.

Nutrition:

Calories:200;

Carbohydrates: 5g;

Protein: 20g;

Fat: 8g;

Sugar: 2g;

Sodium: 594mg;

Fiber: 0g

45. Lemon Sesame Dip

Preparation Time: 10 minutes

Cooking Time: 0 minutes

Servings: 6

Ingredients:

1 cup sesame seed paste

Salt and ground black pepper, to taste

1 cup vegetable stock

½ cup lemon juice

3 garlic cloves, peeled and chopped

2 tablespoons cilantro, chopped

Directions:

In a food processor, mix the sesame seed paste with lemon juice and the other ingredients, pulse, divide into bowls and serve.

Nutrition:

Calories:150;

Carbohydrates: 6.5g;

Protein: 9.4g;

Fat: 5g; Sugar: 1.3g;

Sodium: 254mg;

Fiber: 1.7g

46. Potato Chips

Preparation Time: 10 minutes

Cooking Time: 55 minutes

Servings: 6

Ingredients:

5 bacon slices, cooked and chopped

1 tablespoon fresh rosemary, chopped

3 onions, peeled and chopped

Salt and ground black pepper, to taste

3 dates, pitted and chopped

2 sweet potatoes, sliced

1 tablespoons olive oil + a drizzle

Directions:

Heat a pan with a drizzle of oil over medium heat, add the onions, dates, rosemary, salt and pepper, stir, and cook for 30 minutes stirring often.

Take off the heat, add bacon and stir.

Arrange the potato slices on a baking sheet, add 1 tablespoon oil, toss to coat, bake in the oven at 425°F for 25 minutes, arrange the potato sliced on a platter, top with the bacon mix and serve.

Nutrition:

Calories:190;

Carbohydrates: 12g;

Protein: 17g;

Fat: 3g;

Sugar: 2g;

Sodium: 356mg;

Fiber: 0g

47. Beets Chips

Preparation Time: 1hour 10 minutes

Cooking Time: 30 minutes

Servings: 4

Ingredients:

2 beets, sliced

⅓ cup white vinegar

A pinch of ground black pepper

1 cup olive oil

1 teaspoon green tea powder

Directions:

Put the vinegar in a small pot, heat over medium heat, add tea powder, stir well, bring to a simmer, take off the heat, and cool down.

Add the beets, half of the oil, some black pepper, whisk well and leave aside for 1 hour. Arrange the beets on a lined baking sheet, add the rest of the oil, toss, bake in the oven at 350°F for 30 minutes, divide into bowls and serve.

Nutrition:

Calories:100;

Carbohydrates: 3g;

Protein: 2g;

Fat: 3g;

Sugar: 5g;

Sodium: 574mg;

Fiber: 0g

48. Cabbage Slaw

Preparation Time: 10 minutes

Cooking Time: 0 minutes

Servings: 4

Ingredients:

2 carrots, peeled and grated

1 green cabbage head, shredded

10 strawberries, cored and cut in half

A pinch of salt and black pepper

2 tablespoons white wine vinegar

1 tablespoon Dijon mustard

¼ cup lemon juice

¾ cup olive oil

Directions:

In a bowl, mix the cabbage with the carrots and the other ingredients, toss and serve as an appetizer.

Nutrition:

Calories:100;

Carbohydrates: 2g;

Protein: 4g; Fat: 1g;

Sugar: 3g; Sodium: 540mg;

Fiber: 0g

49. Chicken Bites

Preparation Time: 10 minutes

Cooking Time: 10 minutes

Servings: 4

Ingredients:

20 ounces pineapple slices, cubed

2 teaspoons olive oil

1 tablespoon sweet paprika

3 cups chicken thighs, boneless, skinless, and cut into medium pieces

1 tablespoon parsley, chopped

Directions:

Heat a pan over medium-high heat, add the pineapple slices, grill them for 2 minutes on each side and cool them.

Heat a pan with the oil over medium-high heat, add the chicken and paprika, cook them for 5 minutes on each side, arrange on a platter, top each of the chicken pieces with a pineapple cube, sprinkle the parsley on top, prick with toothpicks and serve.

Nutrition:

Calories:120;

Carbohydrates: 5g;

Protein: 2g;

Fat: 3g;

Sugar: 0g;

Sodium: 254mg;

Fiber: 1.7g

50. Mushroom Platter

Preparation Time: 10 minutes

Cooking Time: 10 minutes

Servings: 6

Ingredients:

8 lemon tea bags

6 Portobello mushroom caps

3 tablespoons cilantro, chopped

A pinch of salt and black pepper

1 cup hot water

1 cup avocado oil

Directions:

In a bowl, mix the water with the tea bags, cover, leave aside for 10 minutes and strain the tea into another bowl. Add the mushrooms and the other ingredients and toss.

Heat a kitchen grill over medium-high heat, add the mushrooms, grill them for 5 minutes on each side, arrange them on a platter and serve.

Nutrition:

Calories:150;

Carbohydrates: 5g;

Protein: 3g;

Fat: 6g;

Sugar: 0.2g;

Sodium: 444mg;

Fiber: 0g

51. Zucchini Spread

Preparation Time: 10 minutes

Cooking Time: 5 minutes

Servings: 6

Ingredients:

2 tablespoons olive oil

2 tablespoons lime juice

2 tablespoons mint leaves, chopped

Ground black pepper, to taste

2 garlic cloves, peeled and minced

4 zucchinis, chopped

½ cup coconut cream

Directions:

Heat a pan with the oil over medium-high heat, add the zucchini and the garlic, stir, cook for 5 minutes, take off the heat and cool down.

In a blender, combine the zucchinis with the remaining ingredients, pulse and serve as a party spread.

Nutrition:

Calories:130;

Carbohydrates: 3g;

Protein: 5g;

Fat: 3g;

Sugar: 0g;

Sodium: 456mg;

Fiber: 0g

Lunch recipes

52. Creamy Cauliflower Risotto

Preparation Time: 15 minutes

Cooking Time: 14 minutes

Servings: 4

Ingredients

- ¼ tsp ground nutmeg
- ¼ cup ghee
- ¼ tsp ground black pepper
- ½ diced onion
- ½ tsp salt
- 1 garlic clove, thinly cut
- 1 cup parmesan cheese, shredded
- 1 head cauliflower, shredded
- ½ cup heavy whipping cream
- 1 cup fresh mushrooms, diced

Directions

Set your stove to medium heat and place a skillet containing the ghee on it. Once the ghee has melted, add garlic and onion. Cook those for 3 minutes, or until you are sure that they are tender.

Next, add the shredded cauliflower and stir for an additional 3 minutes. Also, add your mushrooms and let it cook till tender for, again, 3 minutes. This means that after about 10 minutes of the previous steps, it should be time to add the nutmeg, whipping cream, salt, cheese, and pepper. Continue cooking for about 7 minutes. The content of your skillet should be creamy at this point.

Nutrition:

Calories:; 350

Carbohydrates: 9.8g;

Protein: 12.1g;

Fat: 11g; Sugar: 0.8g;

Sodium: 654mg; Fiber: 2g

53. Spicy Butternut Squash Soup

Preparation Time: 20 minutes

Cooking Time: 35 minutes

Servings: 6

Ingredients

- 1 cup heavy whipping cream
- 1 tbsp extra virgin olive oil
- ½ tsp curry powder
- 1 onion, chopped
- ½ tsp ground ginger
- 2 garlic cloves
- ½ tsp ground black pepper
- 1 lb peeled and seeded butternut squash, thinly cut
- 1 tsp salt
- 5 cups vegetable broth
- 1 tbsp brown sugar

Directions

For this recipe, you'll need a pressure cooker that is multi-functional. Click on saute, before adding the extra virgin olive oil. When the oil is hot, put the diced onion in the cooker and let it saute for 7 minutes. Next, add your garlic and let it cook for 1 minute.

You can add the curry powder, butternut squash, ginger, vegetable broth, ground black pepper, brown sugar, and salt now. Cover the lid of the cooker and secure it. If you have read the manual of the cooker, set it to high pressure. Also, time the build-up of pressure for 1 minutes.

After releasing the pressure with quick release, you can open the lid of the cooker. Releasing the pressure should take all of 5 minutes. Transfer the content of the cooker to a blender and process till you're left with a creamy mixture. Add the heavy whipping cream and stir. Enjoy.

Nutrition: Calories:235;

Carbohydrates: 12.5g;

Protein: 2.4g; Fat: 17.5g;

Sugar: 0.2g; Sodium: 791mg;

Fiber: 4g

54. Cherry Chicken Lettuce Wraps

Preparation Time: 15 minutes

Cooking Time: 10 minutes

Servings: 1

Ingredients

- 12 lettuce leaves
- 2 tbsp canola oil, separated
- ⅓ cup sliced almonds, toasted
- 1 ¼ lb chicken breast, the skin and bones removed and minced
- ½ cup green onion, diced
- 1 tbsp fresh ginger root, thinly cut
- 1 ½ cups carrots, roughly cut
- 2 tbsp rice vinegar
- 1 lb dark sweet cherries, cut in halves and the pits removed
- 2 tbsp teriyaki sauce
- 1 tbsp honey

Directions

Set your stove to medium high heat and place a large sized skillet on it. Add 1 tbsp of oil to the pan and let it get hot. Put the skinless and boneless chicken in the pot and add your ginger. Saute for 10 minutes. Be careful not to burn your chicken. You just want to make sure it is cooked through.

Get a bowl and add honey, vinegar, 1 tbsp oil, and teriyaki sauce. Using a whisk, mix these ingredients well, before throwing in your almonds, the chicken mixture in your skillet, green onion, cherries and carrots.

Using a spoon, place the mixture in the center of each of the twelve lettuce leaves. Roll the lettuce to cover this filling, and they are ready to serve.

Nutrition:

Calories:297;

Carbohydrates: 21.5g;

Protein: 25g;

Fat: 12.4g;

Sugar: 2g;

Sodium: 156mg; Fiber: 1g

55. Easy Korean Beef

Preparation Time: 10 minutes

Cooking Time: 10 minutes

Servings: 4

Ingredients

- 1 tbsp sesame seeds
- 2 tsp sesame oil
- 2 tbsp green onion, diced
- 1 lb lean ground beef
- 2 cups cauliflower rice
- 3 garlic cloves, thinly cut
- ¼ tsp ground black pepper
- ¼ cup soy sauce
- ¼ tsp ground ginger
- 1 tbsp coconut sugar

Directions

Make sure your stove is set to medium high heat and place a large skillet on it. Pour the sesame oil in the pan to make it hot, before adding garlic and ground beef. After 7 minutes, by which time the beef would crumble easily, turn down the stove to low and quickly continue with the next step.

Grab a bowl and throw your black pepper, soy sauce, ginger, and coconut sugar in it. Using a whisk, mix these ingredients properly. Now, you can pour the coconut sugar mixture over the cooked beef that is still in the pan. Increase the heat back to medium and let the beef mixture simmer for about 3 minutes.

Serve the keto korean beef on top of your prepared cauliflower rice. Finally, garnish with sesame seeds and green onions.

Nutrition:

Calories:297;

Carbohydrates: 8.9g;

Protein: 22.4g;

Fat: 13.3g;

Sugar: 0.6g;

Sodium: 956mg;

Fiber: 3.7g

56. Peanut Sesame Shirataki Noodles

Preparation Time: 20 minutes

Cooking Time: 10 minutes

Servings: 4

Ingredients

- 1 8 oz pack shirataki noodles
- 2 tbsp creamy peanut butter
- Snow peas
- 1 tbsp water
- 1 medium carrot, shredded
- 1 tbsp soy sauce, low-sodium
- Peanuts
- 1 tsp rice vinegar
- Toasted sesame seeds
- Pinch garlic powder
- Green onions
- ¼ tsp black pepper
- Cilantro
- 1 tsp brown sugar
- Pinch ground ginger
- ⅛ tsp sesame oil

Directions

Pasta

Grab a medium sized bowl and put the ground ginger, peanut butter, sesame oil, water, brown sugar, soy sauce, black pepper, rice vinegar, and garlic powder inside it. Mix properly and set the bowl aside for 30 minutes.

Next, pop that bowl in the refrigerator until you have to use it on the pasta.

To prepare the pasta

Rinse your shirataki noodles. Follow that by draining the noodles and patting them dry using a paper towel.

Get a nonstick pan and place it over medium low heat. The pan has to be completely dry before the noodles. The purpose of this is to further make sure that the noodles are not wet. Do not burn them.

Chop your snow peas and add them, along with the grated carrots, into the pan containing your noodles. Saute for about 4 minutes before you pour the sauce in. Mix the sauce into the other ingredients well.

Decorate with cilantro, toasted sesame seeds, green onions, and peanuts. Alternatively, you can choose to not garnish the meal.

Nutrition:

Calories:111;

Carbohydrates: 9g;

Protein: 12.6g;

Fat: 6.5g;

Sugar: 1.9g;

Sodium: 564mg;

Fiber: 2g

57. Ginger Asian Slaw

Preparation Time: 15 minutes

Cooking Time: 0 minutes

Servings: 8

Ingredients

- Sea salt to your preferred taste
- 6 cups Napa cabbage, minced
- Pepper to your preferred taste
- 6 cups red cabbage, minced
- 3 tbsp lime juice
- 2 cups carrots grated
- 1 medium lime zest
- 1 cup cilantro, shredded
- ¼ tsp cayenne pepper
- ¾ cup diced green onions
- 1 garlic clove, thinly cut
- 1 tbsp extra virgin olive oil
- 1 ½ inch ginger, shredded
- 1 tbsp maple syrup
- 2 tbsp almond butter
- 1 tsp sesame oil
- 1 tbsp rice vinegar
- 1 tbsp apple cider vinegar
- 2 tbsp tamari

Directions

Into the cup of a blender add your olive oil, salt, pepper, maple syrup, lime juice, sesame oil, lime zest, apple cider vinegar, cayenne pepper, tamari, garlic rice vinegar, ginger, and almond butter. Blend these ingredients until you are left with a smooth mixture. This is your dressing.

Next, you'll need a large mixing bowl. Put the cilantro, cabbage, green onions, and carrots inside it. Pour the mixture in your blender into the bowl and toss well.

For about an hour, let the bowl stay in your fridge. The various flavors will meld deliciously and afterwards, you can serve.

Nutrition:

Calories:144;

Carbohydrates: 12g;

Protein: 24.4g;

Fat: 6g;

Sugar: 1.7g;

Sodium: 432mg;

Fiber: 1.7g

58. Zucchini Cream

Preparation Time: 10 minutes

Cooking Time: 25 minutes

Servings: 8

Ingredients: 4 cups vegetable stock -2 tablespoons olive oil

2 sweet potatoes, peeled and cubed

8 zucchinis, chopped

2 onions, peeled and chopped

1 cup coconut milk

A pinch of salt and black pepper

1 teaspoon dried rosemary

4 tablespoons fresh dill, chopped - ½ teaspoon fresh basil, chopped

Directions: Heat a pot with the oil over medium heat, add the onion, stir, and cook for 2 minutes. Add the zucchinis and the rest of the ingredients except the milk and dill, stir and simmer for 20 minutes.

Add the milk and dill, puree the soup using an immersion blender, stir, ladle into soup bowls and serve.

Nutrition: Calories:324;

Carbohydrates: 10g;

Protein: 14.8g; Fat: 3g;

Sugar: 1.8g; Sodium: 585mg;

Fiber: 0.4g

59. Chicken Soup

Preparation Time: 10 minutes

Cooking Time: 20 minutes

Servings: 4

Ingredients:

4 cups vegetable stock

1 lemongrass stalk, chopped

1 small ginger piece, peeled and grated

A pinch of salt and black pepper

12 ounces coconut milk

1 pound chicken breast, skinless, boneless, and cut into thin strips

8 ounces mushrooms, chopped

4 Serrano chilies, chopped

4 tablespoons coconut aminos

¼ cup lime juice

¼ cup fresh parsley, chopped

Directions:

Put the stock into a pot, add the lemongrass and ginger, stir, and cook over medium heat for 10 minutes. Strain this mix into another pot, heat over medium, add the chicken and the rest of the ingredients, stir, simmer for 10 minutes, ladle into bowls, and serve.

Nutrition:

Calories:150;

Carbohydrates: 4g;

Protein: 20.4g;

Fat: 6g;

Sugar: 2g;

Sodium: 623mg;

Fiber: 0.3g

60. Paprika Turkey Burgers

Preparation Time: 10 minutes

Cooking Time: 10 minutes

Servings: 4

Ingredients:

 1 pound ground turkey

Zest of 1 lime, grated

2 teaspoons lime juice

1 shallot, peeled and minced

3 teaspoons olive oil

1 jalapeño pepper, minced

Salt and ground black pepper, to taste

1 teaspoon cumin

1-teaspoon paprika

Directions:

In a bowl, mix the turkey meat lime zest and the other ingredients except the oil, stir and shape 4 burgers out of this mix. Heat a pan with the oil over medium-high heat, add the turkey burgers, cook them for 4-5 minutes on each side, divide between plates and serve.

Nutrition:

Calories:200;

Carbohydrates: 0.4g;

Protein: 29.4g;

Fat: 12g;

Sugar: 1g;

Sodium: 543mg;

Fiber: 0g

61. Turkey and Broccoli Soup

Preparation Time: 15 minutes

Cooking Time: 35 minutes

Servings: 4

Ingredients:

4 shallots, peeled and chopped

3 carrots, peeled and chopped

1 pound turkey, ground

6 cups chicken stock

Salt and ground black pepper, to taste

1 red bell pepper, seeded and chopped

2 cups broccoli florets, chopped

4 cups kale, chopped

2 tablespoons coconut oil

15 ounces canned diced tomatoes

Directions:

Heat a pot with the oil over medium-high heat, add the shallots, broccoli, carrots and bell pepper, stir, and cook for 10 minutes.

Add the turkey and the other ingredients, stir, reduce heat, simmer soup for 25 minutes, ladle into bowls and serve.

Nutrition:

Calories:150;

Carbohydrates: 4g;

Protein: 6g;

Fat: 4g;

Sugar: 1g;

Sodium: 654mg;

Fiber: 0.8g

62. Wrapped Asparagus

Preparation Time: 10 minutes

Cooking Time: 10 minutes

Servings: 4

Ingredients:

1 pound asparagus, trimmed

1 tablespoon olive oil

1 teaspoon sweet paprika

Salt and ground black pepper, to taste

A pinch of garlic powder

4 ounces smoked salmon

Directions:

Put the asparagus spears on a lined baking sheet, drizzle the oil, season with salt, pepper, paprika, garlic powder, rub and roast in the oven at 390 ° F for 15 minutes.

Wrap 4 asparagus spears in 1 ounce smoked salmon, repeat with the rest of the asparagus, put the wraps on a lined baking sheet, broil over medium high heat for 3 minutes, divide between plates and serve.

Nutrition:

Calories:90;

Carbohydrates: 1.5g;

Protein: 23.4g;

Fat: 5g;

Sugar: 2g;

Sodium: 309mg;

Fiber: 0.5g

63. Salmon and Lemon Sauce

Preparation Time: 10 minutes

Cooking Time: 20 minutes

Servings: 4

Ingredients:

4 salmon fillets, boneless

3 garlic cloves, peeled and minced

1 onion, peeled and chopped

Salt and ground black pepper, to taste

2 tablespoons olive oil

¼ cup fresh parsley, chopped

Juice of 1 lemon

1 lemon, sliced

1 tablespoon fresh thyme, chopped

4 cups water

Directions:

Heat a pan with the oil over medium-high heat, add the onion and garlic, salt and pepper stir, and cook for 5 minutes.

Add the salmon, parsley and the other ingredients, toss gently, cook for 15 minutes, divide between plates and serve.

Nutrition:

Calories:133;

Carbohydrates: 4g;

Protein: 24g;

Fat: 8g;

Sugar: 2g;

Sodium: 608mg;

Fiber: 0.4g

64. Beef Salad

Preparation Time: 10 minutes

Cooking Time: 15 minutes

Servings: 4

Ingredients:

2 tomatoes, cored and chopped

2 avocados, pitted and chopped

6 cups romaine lettuce leaves, chopped

1 onion, peeled and chopped

Juice of 2 limes

1 pound ground beef

2 garlic cloves, peeled and minced

1 teaspoon cumin

2 teaspoons olive oil

Salt and ground black pepper, to taste

1 bunch fresh cilantro, chopped

2 teaspoons chili powder

Directions:

Heat a pan with the oil over medium-high heat, add the onion, stir, and cook for 5 minutes.

Add the garlic, salt, pepper, chili powder, cumin and the beef, stir, and cook for 10 minutes.

In a salad bowl, mix the beef with all the other ingredients, toss and serve.

Nutrition:

Calories:143;

Carbohydrates: 12g;

Protein: 9g;

Fat: 6g; Sugar: 0.1g;

Sodium: 752mg;

Fiber: 0g

65. Sausage Mix

Preparation Time: 10 minutes

Cooking Time: 15 minutes

Servings: 2

Ingredients:

1 pound sausage, casings removed and chopped

1 tomato, cubed

1 onion, peeled and chopped

1 bunch kale, chopped

Salt and ground black pepper, to taste

Directions:

Heat a pan over medium-high heat; add the sausage meat, stir, and brown for 5 minutes.

Add the rest of the ingredients, toss, cook for 10 minutes more, divide into bowls and serve.

Nutrition:

Calories:170;

Carbohydrates: 10g;

Protein: 12g;

Fat: 3g; Sugar: 0.4g;

Sodium: 650mg;

Fiber: 0.5g

66. Garlic Burgers

Preparation Time: 10 minutes

Cooking Time: 10 minutes

Servings: 7

Ingredients: ½ pound bacon, minced - 1½ pounds ground beef - A drizzle of olive oil

Salt and ground black pepper, to taste

6 garlic cloves, peeled and minced

Directions: *In a bowl, mix the beef with the bacon, garlic, salt, and pepper, stir well and shape medium patties from this mixture.*

Heat a pan with the oil over medium-high heat, add the burgers, cook them for about 5 minutes, flip, cook for 5 more minutes, divide between plates and serve with a side salad.

Nutrition: Calories:200;

Carbohydrates: 12g;

Protein: 14g; Fat: 5g;

Sugar: 2g; Sodium: 480mg;

Fiber: 1g

67. Sweet Potato Casserole

Preparation Time: 10 minutes

Cooking Time: 1 hour

Servings: 4

Ingredients:

2½ tablespoons olive oil

2 cups sweet potatoes, grated

6 eggs

A drizzle of olive oil

5 bacon slices, cooked and crumbled

Salt and ground black pepper, to taste

8 cherry tomatoes, cut in quarters

1 small onion, peeled and chopped

½ cup arugula leaves

3 garlic cloves, peeled and minced

Directions:

Arrange the sweet potatoes in a baking dish and bake in the oven at 450°F for 20 minutes.

Heat a pan with the oil over medium heat, add the onions, stir, and cook for 5 minutes. ·

Add the arugula, the garlic and tomatoes, stir, cook for 5 minutes and add over the potatoes.

Also add the whisked eggs and the rest of the ingredients, bake in the oven at 350°F for 30 minutes and serve hot.

Nutrition:

Calories:215;

Carbohydrates: 4g;

Protein: 9g;

Fat: 9g;

Sugar: 1g;

Sodium: 801mg;

Fiber: 0g

68. Sausage and Tomato Muffins

Preparation Time: 25 minutes

Cooking Time: 10 minutes

Servings: 12

Ingredients:

2 garlic cloves, peeled and minced

¾ pound sausage, casings removed

Salt and ground black pepper, to taste

⅔ cup sun-dried tomatoes, chopped

1 teaspoon onion powder

10 eggs

2 teaspoons olive oil

Directions:

Heat a pan with the oil over medium-high heat, add the sausage and brown for 5 minutes.

Add the garlic and the tomatoes, stir and cook for 5 minutes.

Combine with the eggs and the rest of the ingredients, stir, divide this into a greased muffin tray, bake in the oven at 400°F for 15 minutes and serve.

Nutrition:

Calories:321;

Carbohydrates: 8g;

Protein: 10.2g;

Fat: 9g;

Sugar: 3g;

Sodium: 350mg;

Fiber: 1.7g

69. Sweet Potato Salad

Preparation Time: 10 minutes

Cooking Time: 10 minutes

Servings: 3

Ingredients:

2 teaspoons olive oil

1 sweet potato, spiralized

1 apple, cored and spiralized

3 tablespoons almonds, toasted and sliced

Salt, to taste

3 cups spinach, torn

For the salad dressing:

1 teaspoon apple cider vinegar

2 tablespoons apple juice

1 tablespoon almond butter, melted

½ teaspoon ginger, minced

1½ teaspoons mustard

1 tablespoon olive oil

Directions:

In a bowl, mix the vinegar with the apple juice, almond butter, ginger, mustard and 1 tablespoon oil and whisk.

Heat a pan with the 2 teaspoons oil over medium-high heat, add the sweet potato noodles, stir, cook for 7 minutes and transfer to a bowl.

Add the rest of the ingredients and the dressing, toss and serve.

Nutrition: Calories:500;

Carbohydrates: 7g;

Protein: 8g; Fat: 2g; Sugar: 0.3g;

Sodium: 434mg; Fiber: 0g

70. Cauliflower Salad

Preparation Time: 10 minutes

Cooking Time: 0 minutes

Servings: 4

Ingredients:

2 tablespoons olive oil

1 cup black olives, pitted and halved

6 cups cauliflower florets, grated and blanched

Salt and ground black pepper, to taste

¼ cup onion, chopped

1 teaspoon fresh mint leaves, chopped

1 tablespoon fresh parsley, chopped

Juice of ½ lemon

Directions:

In a salad bowl, mix the cauliflower with the olives and the other ingredients, toss and serve.

Nutrition:

Calories:860;

Carbohydrates: 6g;

Protein: 10.5g;

Fat: 6g;

Sugar: 1g;

Sodium: 604mg;

Fiber: 1g

Pork Recipes

71. Pesto Pork Roast

Preparation Time: 30 minutes

Cooking Time:1hour 30 minutes

Servings: 8

Ingredients

1/4 cup plus 2 tbsps. olive oil, divided

2 cups loosely packed basil leaves

1/2 cup grated Parmesan cheese

4 garlic cloves, peeled

12 plum tomatoes

1-1/2 **tsps.** pepper, divided

1 **tsp.** kosher salt, divided

1 bone-in pork loin roast (4 to 5 **lbs.**)

1 package (16 **oz.**) egg noodles

Directions

To make pesto, combine garlic, cheese, basil, and 1/4 cup oil in a blender, put on the lid and puree until smooth. Take 2 **tbsps.** of pesto sauce and put into a small bowl; mix in the remainder of oil; put aside.

Divide each tomato into 4 slices; arrange tomato slices in a greased shallow roasting pan. Sprinkle with 1/2 **tsp.** salt and 1 **tsp.** pepper to season.

Sprinkle the remaining salt and pepper over the roast; position roast atop slices of tomatoes. Distribute the remaining pesto over the roast.

Bake without covering for 1.5 to 2 hours at 350° until a thermometer registers 160°.

Take roast out of the oven; keep warm. Allow roast to rest for 10 minutes before cutting. In the meantime, cook noodles as directed on package; drain; transfer to a large bowl.

Add tomatoes to noodles using a slotted spoon; toss in the reserved pesto sauce until well combined. Serve noodles with pork

Nutrition:

Calories:584;

Carbohydrates: 26g;

Protein: 43g;

Fat: 25g;

Sugar: 2.2g;

Sodium: 426mg;

Fiber: 3g

72. Pork Roast with Fruit Sauce

Preparation Time: 25 minutes

Cooking Time: 2hours 25 minutes

Servings: 12

Ingredients

1 bone-in pork loin roast (3 to 4 **lbs.**)

1 jar (10 **oz.**) apple jelly

1 cup apple juice

1/2 **tsp.** ground cardamom

3/4 cup chopped dried apricots

1 **tbsp.** cornstarch

2 **tbsps.** water

Direction

Arrange roast on a rack in a shallow roasting pan. Bake without a cover for 1 hour and 30 minutes at 350°.

Combine cardamom, apple juice, and apple jelly in a saucepan; cook over medium heat until thoroughly heated and smooth, stirring well. Measure 1/2 cup sauce and set aside. Brush roast evenly with some of the remaining sauce.

Bake until a thermometer registers 160°, for 40 to 60 minutes, brushing roast with sauce after each 20 minutes.

Transfer roast to a serving platter; keep warm. Transfer pan juices into a saucepan.

Add reserved fruit sauce and apricots. Cook for about 5 minutes over medium heat until softened. Stir together water and cornstarch until smooth; add into apricot mixture.

Cook, stirring, about 2 minutes, until boiling. Serve roast with sauce.

Nutrition:

Calories:233;

Carbohydrates: 24g;

Protein: 22g;

Fat: 5g;

Sugar: 0.3g;

Sodium: 504mg;

Fiber: 1.6g

73. Carolina-style Pork Barbecue

Preparation Time: 30 minutes

Cooking Time:6hours 30 minutes

Servings: 14

Ingredients

1 boneless pork shoulder butt roast (4 to 5 **lbs.**)

2 **tbsps.** brown sugar

2 **tsps.** salt

1 **tsp.** paprika

1/2 **tsp.** pepper

2 medium onions, quartered

3/4 cup cider vinegar

4 **tsps.** Worcestershire sauce

1 **tbsp.** sugar

1 **tbsp.** crushed red pepper flakes

1 **tsp.** garlic salt

1 **tsp.** ground mustard

1/2 **tsp.** cayenne pepper

14 hamburger buns, split

1-3/4 **lbs.** deli coleslaw

Direction

Quarter the roast.

Mix pepper, paprika, salt, and brown sugar; rub on the meat.

Arrange onion and meat in a 5-quart slow cooker.

Whisk seasonings, sugar, Worcestershire sauce, and vinegar in a small bowl; spread over the roast. Cook, covered, for 6 to 8 hours on low until meat is softened.

Transfer the roast; let cool slightly. Save 1 1/2 cups of cooking juices; discard the leftover juices. Skim the grease from reserved juices. With 2 forks, shred the pork.

Bring the reserved juices and pork back to the slow cooker; heat through. Serve with coleslaw on buns.

Nutrition:

Calories:400;

Carbohydrates: 25g;

Protein: 27g;

Fat: 34g;

Sugar: 2g;

Sodium: 490mg;

Fiber: 0g

74. Slow-cooked Pork And Beans

Preparation Time: 15 minutes

Cooking Time: 15 minutes

Servings: 12

Ingredients

1 boneless pork loin roast (3 **lbs.**)

1 medium onion, sliced

3 cans (15 **oz.** each) pork and beans

1-1/2 cups barbecue sauce

1/4 cup packed brown sugar

1 **tsp.** garlic powder

Direction

Slice the roast into 2 equal parts and put in a 5-qt. slow cooker. Put onion on top. Combine garlic powder, brown sugar, barbecue sauce, and beans in a large bowl; pour over the meat. Cover and cook on low until the meat is soft, or for 6-8 hours. Remove the roast; use 2 forks to shred. Bring the meat back to the slow cooker and heat through

Nutrition: Calories:217;

Carbohydrates: 4g;

Protein: 24g; Fat: 6g;

Sugar: 2.2g; Sodium: 507mg;

Fiber: 2g

75. Chipotle Pomegranate Pulled Pork

Preparation Time: 10 minutes

Cooking Time: 40 minutes

Servings: 10

Ingredients

1 boneless pork shoulder butt roast (3 **lbs.**)

2 **tbsps.** steak seasoning

1/2 cup water

1 half-pint jar Pomegranate Jelly or 1 cup red currant jelly

3 **tbsps.** minced chipotle peppers in adobo sauce

10 kaiser rolls, split

Direction

Halve the roast and put into a 5-quart slow cooker, then sprinkle steak seasoning over top.

Put in water and cook with a cover on low setting until roast is tender, about 8 to 10 hours.

Mix peppers and jelly together in a small saucepan, then cook on moderate heat until heated through, about 5 minutes.

Take the meat out of slow cooker and get rid of cooking liquid. Use 2 forks to shred the pork and turn back the slow cooker.

Put jelly mixture on top then place a cover and cook on low setting until heated through, about half an hour. Scoop each roll with 2/3 cup meat.

Nutrition:

Calories:678;

Carbohydrates: 20g;

Protein: 37g;

Fat: 28g;

Sugar: 3g;

Sodium: 839mg;

Fiber: 1g

76. Apple Roasted Pork With Cherry Balsamic Glaze

Preparation Time: 30 minutes

Cooking Time: 1hour 20 minutes

Servings: 8

Ingredients

1 boneless pork loin roast (3 **lbs.**)

1-1/2 **tsps.** salt, divided

3/4 **tsp.** pepper, divided

1/4 cup olive oil, divided

3 medium apples, sliced

1-1/2 cups unsweetened apple juice

6 medium onions, sliced (about 5 cups)

3 **tbsps.** balsamic vinegar

1-1/2 cups frozen pitted dark sweet cherries

1/2 cup cherry juice

Direction

Set the oven to 350° to preheat. Season the roast with 1/2 **tsp.** of pepper and 1 **tsp.** of salt.

Heat 2 **tbsps.** oil in an ovenproof Dutch oven over medium-high heat; cook all sides of the roast until browned. Add apple juice and apples to pan. Bake without a cover while basting occasionally with pan juices for 50-60 minutes, until a thermometer shows 145° when inserted in pork.

In the meantime, heat the leftover oil in a large skillet over medium heat.

Put in the onions and the leftover salt and pepper; cook while stirring for 8-10 minutes, until tender. Lower the heat to medium-low; continue to cook while stirring occasionally for 35-40 minutes until it turns deep golden brown. Keep warm.

Transfer apples and roast to a serving plate; cover with foil. Allow the roast to sit for 10 minutes before cutting.

Skim off the fat from pork pan juices. Put over medium-high heat; put in vinegar and cook while stirring to loosen browned bits from pan for 1 minute. Stir in cherry juice and cherries.

Heat to a boil; cook for 10-15 minutes more, until the mixture's volume reduces to about 1 cup. Serve pork, onions and apples along with cherry glaze.

Nutrition:

Calories:387;

Carbohydrates: 29g;

Protein: 34g;

Fat: 15g;

Sugar: 1g;

Sodium: 304mg;

Fiber: 3g

77. Orange-maple Pork Roast

Preparation Time: 20 minutes

Cooking Time: 1hour 50 minutes

Servings: 14

Ingredients

1 can (11 **oz.**) mandarin oranges

1 boneless whole pork loin roast (about 4 **lbs.**)

2 **tbsps.** olive oil

1/2 cup maple syrup

2 **tbsps.** minced fresh rosemary or 2 **tsps.** dried rosemary, crushed

Sliced starfruit

Direction

Drain oranges, reserving the juice; set oranges and juice aside.

Brown roast in a large skillet with hot oil on all sides.

Place on a rack in a shallow roasting pan.

Mix the reserved juice and syrup together; transfer over the roast. Sprinkle rosemary over.

Bake with a cover at 325° for 1 1/2-2 hours, basting every 30 minutes, or till a thermometer reads 160°.

Allow to stand for 10-15 minutes before slicing.

Use the reserved oranges and starfruit for garnish. Drizzle with pan juices if you want.

Nutrition:

Calories:194;

Carbohydrates: 10g;

Protein: 22g;

Fat: 7g;

Sugar: 0.2g;

Sodium: 125mg;

Fiber: 0g

78. Moist Cranberry Pork Roast

Preparation Time: 5 minutes

Cooking Time: 4hour 05 minutes

Servings: 8

Ingredients

1 boneless rolled pork loin roast (2-1/2 to 3 **lbs.**)

1/2 **tsp.** salt

1/4 **tsp.** pepper

1 can (14 **oz.**) whole-berry cranberry sauce

1/4 cup honey

1 **tsp.** grated orange zest

1/8 **tsp.** ground cloves

1/8 **tsp.** ground nutmeg

Direction

Divide roast in 2 equal portions; arrange in a 3-quart slow cooker; season roasts with pepper and salt. Mix remaining ingredients together; pour over roast in the cooker.

Cook on low setting, covered, until a thermometer registers 160°, for 4 to 5 hours.

Allow to rest for 10 minutes before serving.

Nutrition:

Calories:290;

Carbohydrates: 8.5g;

Protein: 23g;

Fat: 6g;

Sugar: 2.1g;

Sodium: 201mg;

Fiber: 1g

79. Homemade Marinated Pork Roast

Preparation Time: 15 minutes

Cooking Time: 2hours

Servings: 6

Ingredients

1 liter ginger ale

1/2 cup soy sauce

1/4 cup finely chopped green pepper

4 garlic cloves, minced

1 **tbsp.** lemon juice

1 **tbsp.** sugar

1 bone-in center cut pork roast (3 to 4 **lbs.**)

1/4 cup all-purpose flour

1/3 cup water

Direction

In one big heavy-duty resealable plastic bag or shallow glass dish, mix the initial six ingredients.

Put in the pork roast. Seal or cover and keep in the refrigerator overnight, flipping one time.

Add the marinade and roast into the shallow roasting pan.

Bake at 325 degrees till the thermometer reaches 160 to 170 degrees or for 1 hour and 45 minutes. Allow it to rest for 10 minutes.

At the same time, measure 2 cups pan of the drippings.

Skim off fat; add to the sauce pan. Mix water and flour till smooth; put into the drippings.

Boil; cook and whisk for 2 minutes.

Serve along with roast.

Nutrition:

Calories:250;

Carbohydrates: 17g;

Protein: 29g;

Fat: 8g;

Sugar: 3.1g;

Sodium: 987mg;

Fiber: 0g

80. Pork 'n' Pepper Tortillas

Preparation Time: 20 minutes

Cooking Time: 8hours 20 minutes

Servings: 12

Ingredients

1 boneless pork shoulder butt roast (3 **lbs.**), halved

1 cup boiling water

2 **tsps.** beef bouillon granules

3 garlic cloves, minced

1 **tbsp.** dried basil

1 **tbsp.** dried oregano

1 **tsp.** ground cumin

1 **tsp.** pepper

1 **tsp.** dried tarragon

1 **tsp.** white pepper

2 medium onions, sliced

1 each large green, sweet red and yellow peppers, sliced

1 **tbsp.** butter

12 flour tortillas (8 inches), warmed

Shredded lettuce, chopped ripe olives, sliced jalapeno peppers and sour cream, optional

Direction

Put the roast in a 5-quart slow cooker.

Combine seasonings, garlic, bouillon, and water; pour over the roast. Top with onions.

Cover and cook on high for 1 hour.

Lower the heat to low. Cook for 7 to 8 hours until pork is very tender.

Take out the meat; shred with 2 forks. Bring back to slow

cooker; heat through. In the meantime, sauté peppers in butter in a skillet until tender. With a slotted spoon, put about 1/2 cup of pork and onion mixture down the center of each tortilla; top with peppers. Top with your favorite toppings, if wanted. Fold sides of tortilla over the filling; serve immediately.

Nutrition:

Calories:470;

Carbohydrates: 19g;

Protein: 36g;

Fat: 6g;

Sugar: 2.2g;

Sodium: 489mg;

Fiber: 0.3g

81. Citrus-herb Pork Roast

Preparation Time: 25 minutes

Cooking Time: 4hours 25 minutes

Servings: 8

Ingredients

1 boneless pork sirloin roast (3 to 4 **lbs.**)

1 **tsp.** dried oregano

1/2 **tsp.** ground ginger

1/2 **tsp.** pepper

2 medium onions, cut into thin wedges

1 cup plus 3 **tbsps.** orange juice, divided

1 **tbsp.** sugar

1 **tbsp.** white grapefruit juice

1 **tbsp.** steak sauce

1 **tbsp.** reduced-sodium soy sauce

1 **tsp.** grated orange zest

1/2 **tsp.** salt

3 **tbsps.** cornstarch

Hot cooked egg noodles

Minced fresh oregano, optional

Direction

Halve roast. Mix pepper, ginger and oregano in a small bowl; rub over pork.

Brown roast on all the sides in a big nonstick skillet coated with cooking spray.

Put into a 4-qt. slow cooker then add onions.

Mix soy sauce, steak sauce, grapefruit juice, sugar and 1 cup orange juice in a small bowl; put over the top.

Cover; cook till meat is tender for 4-5 hours on low. Put onions and meat on a serving platter and keep warm.

From cooking juices, skim fat; put into a small saucepan.

Add salt and orange zest; boil. Mix leftover orange juice and cornstarch till smooth; mix into the pan slowly.

Boil; mix and cook till thickened for 2 minutes.

Serve with noodles and pork; sprinkle with fresh oregano, if desired.

Nutrition:

Calories:289;

Carbohydrates: 13g;

Protein: 35g;

Fat: 10g;

Sugar: 1g;

Sodium: 326mg;

Fiber: 0g

82. Asian Barbecued Pork Loin

Preparation Time: 15 minutes

Cooking Time:1hour 15 minutes

Servings: 8

Ingredients

1 boneless whole pork loin roast (3 to 4 **lbs.**)

1/2 **tsp.** garlic salt

1/4 **tsp.** pepper

1/4 cup finely chopped onion

1 **tbsp.** butter

1/2 cup ketchup

1/3 cup honey

1 **tbsp.** hoisin sauce

1-1/2 **tsps.** Chinese-style mustard

1 **tsp.** reduced-sodium soy sauce

1/2 **tsp.** garlic powder

1/4 **tsp.** ground ginger

1/4 **tsp.** Chinese five-spice powder

Direction

Scatter pepper and garlic salt on pork roast.

Add into the shallow roasting pan that is lined with the heavy-duty foil. Bake, with no cover, at 350 degrees for 50 minutes.

At the same time, in a small-sized sauce pan, sauté the onion in butter till soft.

Whisk in rest of the ingredients. Boil. Lower the heat; let simmer, with no cover, for roughly 20 to 25 minutes or till the sauce decrease to three quarters cup, whisking frequently.

Brush the sauce on pork. Bake till the thermometer reaches 145 degrees or for 10 to 15 more minutes. Allow it to rest for 10 minutes prior to slicing.

Nutrition:

Calories:232;

Carbohydrates: 14g;

Protein: 29.4g;

Fat: 6g;

Sugar: 0.2g;

Sodium: 348mg;

Fiber: 0g

83. Conga Lime Pork

Preparation Time: 20 minutes

Cooking Time:4hours 20 minutes

Servings: 6

Ingredients

1 **tsp.** salt, divided

1/2 **tsp.** pepper, divided

1 boneless pork shoulder butt roast (2 to 3 **lbs.**)

1 **tbsp.** canola oil

1 large onion, chopped

3 garlic cloves, peeled and thinly sliced - 1/2 cup water

2 chipotle peppers in adobo sauce, seeded and chopped

2 **tbsps.** molasses

2 cups broccoli coleslaw mix

1 medium mango, peeled and chopped

2 **tbsps.** lime juice

1-1/2 **tsps.** grated lime zest

6 prepared corn muffins, halved

Lime wedges, optional

Direction Sprinkle the roast with 1/4 **tsp.** of pepper and 3/4 **tsp.** of salt. Brown the pork in hot oil on all sides in a large skillet. Place the meat to a 3- or 4-quart slow cooker. In the same skillet, sauté onion until softened. Add garlic; cook for an additional 1 minute. Add molasses, chipotle peppers, and water, stirring to loosen browned bits from pan. Spread over the pork. Cover and cook on high until meat is tender for 4 to 5 hours.

Transfer the roast; let cool slightly. Skim the grease from cooking juices.

With 2 forks, shred the pork and bring back to the slow cooker; heat through.

Combine the remaining pepper and salt, lime zest, lime juice, mango, and coleslaw mix in a large bowl.

Arrange muffin halves with the cut side down on an ungreased baking sheet.

Broil 4-inch away from the heat until lightly toasted for 2 to 3 minutes. Serve with lime wedges, if wanted, and muffins; pour the slaw on top.

Nutrition: Calories:514;

Carbohydrates: 16g;

Protein: 21g; Fat: 6g; Sugar: 3g;

Sodium: 877mg; Fiber: 1.7g

84. Spiced Apple Pork Roast

Preparation Time: 10 minutes

Cooking Time:2hours 10 minutes

Servings: 12

Ingredients

1 boneless rolled pork loin roast (4 to 5 **lbs.**), trimmed

1 garlic clove, cut into lengthwise strips

2 **tbsps.** all-purpose flour

1 **tsp.** prepared mustard

1 **tsp.** salt

1/2 **tsp.** sugar

1/8 **tsp.** pepper

1 cup applesauce

1/3 cup packed brown sugar

2 **tsps.** vinegar

1/8 to 1/4 **tsp.** ground cloves

Direction

Make slits in top of roast; insert garlic strips. Mix pepper, sugar, salt, mustard and flour; rub over the roast. Arrange it fat side up on a rack in a roasting pan.

Bake without a cover at 325° till a thermometer reads 160°, about 2-2 1/2 hours.

Mix cloves, vinegar, brown sugar and applesauce; generously brush over the roast during the last half an hour of baking.

Allow to sit for 10 minutes before slicing.

Nutrition:

Calories:180;

Carbohydrates: 88g;

Protein: 23g;

Fat: 6g;

Sugar: 0.5g;

Sodium: 198mg;

Fiber: 0g

85. Roast Pork and Potatoes

Preparation Time: 20 minutes

Cooking Time: 2hours 50 minutes

Servings: 8

Ingredients

1 envelope onion soup mix

2 garlic cloves, minced

1 **tbsp.** dried rosemary, crushed

1/2 **tsp.** salt

1/2 **tsp.** pepper

1/4 **tsp.** ground cloves

3 cups water, divided

1 bone-in pork loin roast (4 to 5 **lbs.**)

2 to 3 **lbs.** small red potatoes, cut in half

1-1/2 cups sliced onions

Direction

Mix the first 6 ingredients together in a large bowl.

Mix in a half cup of water; allow to sit for 3 minutes.

Place roast on a greased rack in a roasting pan, fat side up.

Pour the remaining water into the pan. Combine onions and potatoes; spread all over the roast. Brush seasoning mixture evenly over roast and vegetables.

Bake without covering for 2.5 to 3 hours at 325°, basting and stirring potatoes sometimes, until a thermometer registers 160° and potatoes are softened. Cover roast with aluminum foil if it's getting brown too quickly. Thicken pan juices for gravy if desired. Allow roast to rest for 10 minutes before slicing.

Nutrition:

Calories:280;

Carbohydrates: 21g;

Protein: 29g;

Fat: 9g;

Sugar: 1.1g;

Sodium: 434mg;

Fiber: 3g

Lamp Recipes

86. Lamb Rack With Cucumber Yogurt

Preparation Time: 25 minutes

Cooking Time: 1hour 45 minutes

Servings: 4

Ingredients

1 1/2 cups plain Greek-style yogurt

2 cucumbers

Salt

2 tsps. lemon juice

1 tbsp. olive oil

1/2 clove garlic

1 1/2 tbsps. chopped dill

1 tbsp. canola oil

1 lamb rack (about 2 1/4 lbs.), frenched and tied

Salt

2 tbsps. butter

5 sprigs thyme

1 clove garlic, crushed but kept whole

Direction

Cucumber yogurt: Line quadruple cheesecloth layer on a colander; put yogurt into cheesecloth. Suspend above a big bowl; refrigerate, letting moisture drain from yogurt, for 48 hours.

Peel then grate cucumbers on box grater; season using 1 tsp. salt. To drain extra moisture, hand for 1 hour in quadruple cheesecloth layer. Get 1 cup drained yogurt; put leftover aside for another time.

Mix drained cucumbers and 1 cup yogurt in a medium bowl; mix in olive oil and lemon juice. Grate garlic on Microplane grater into mixture; fold in chopped dill. Stir well; season to taste with salt.Roasted lamb rack: Preheat an oven to 300°F.

Heat big cast-iron skillet on high heat. Generously use salt to season lamb rack. Put rack, fat side down, in skillet; sear on high heat for 2 1/2-3 minutes till browned. Flip; sear bottom for 1 minute. Flip rack onto fat side; add garlic, thyme and butter. Baste rack for 2 1/2-3 minutes with butter. Put lamb rack onto wire rack in rimmed baking sheet, fat side up; roast for 10 minutes in oven. Flip rack; baste with butter. Put in oven for 10 minutes. Take lamb rack from oven; flip. Baste again. Roast in oven till internal temperature is 130-135°F for 10-15 minutes. Rest lamb rack before slicing for 10-15 minutes. Serve with heirloom tomatoes and cucumber yogurt. Nutrition:Calories:928;Fat: 83g; Carbohydrates: 11g; Sugar: 0.5g; Protein: 36g; Sodium: 1247mg; Fiber: 0g

87. Keto Rack Of Lamb

Preparation Time: 15 minutes

Cooking Time: 45 minutes

Servings: 4

Ingredients

2 racks of lamb (1-1/2 lbs. each)

1/4 cup grated lemon zest

1/4 cup minced fresh oregano or 4 tsps. dried oregano

6 garlic cloves, minced

1 tbsp. olive oil

1/4 tsp. salt

1/4 tsp. pepper

Fresh oregano and lemon slices, optional

Direction

Preheat an oven to 375°. In a shallow roasting pan, put lamb. Mix pepper, salt, oil, garlic, oregano and lemon zest in small bowl; rub over lamb.

Bake for 30-40 minutes till meat gets desired doneness (thermometer should read 145° for medium well; 140° for medium and 135° for medium rare). Before cutting, stand for 5 minutes; serve with lemon slices and fresh oregano if desired.

Nutrition:

Calories:307;

Carbohydrates: 3g;

Protein: 30g;

Fat: 19g;

Sugar: 0.2g;

Sodium: 241mg;

Fiber: 1.7g

88. Mustard And Herb Crusted Rack Of Lamb

Preparation Time: 25 minutes

Cooking Time: 40 minutes

Servings: 8

Ingredients

1 1/2 cups fine fresh bread crumbs

3 tbsps. finely chopped fresh flat-leaf parsley

1 tbsp. finely chopped fresh mint

1 1/2 tsps. minced fresh rosemary

1/2 tsp. salt

1/4 tsp. black pepper

3 1/2 tbsps. olive oil

3 frenched racks of lamb (8 ribs and 1 1/2 lb each rack), trimmed of all but a thin layer of fat, then brought to room temperature

2 tbsps. Dijon mustard

an instant-read thermometer

Direction

Mix together the parsley, salt, rosemary, mint, bread crumbs, and pepper in the bowl. Drizzle with 2 1/2 tbsps. of oil and toss to blend well.

Set oven to 400°F and position oven rack at the center.

Season the lamb with pepper and salt. On moderately high heat, place a large heavy skillet and heat the remaining tbsp. of oil until hot but not smoking. Brown the lamb 1 rack at a time, flipping once, about 4 minutes on each rack. Prepare a 13x9x2 inch roasting pan and place browned lamb; arrange with the fatty sides up.

Spread 2 tsps. of mustard on each rack with fatty sides. In 3 portions, distribute the bread crumbs and per portion, pat over coating each rack with mustard. Press slowly to stick.

Roast lamb until a thermometer inserted diagonally 2 inches at the middle shows 130°F (medium-rare) for 20-25 minutes. Prepare a chopping board; transfer roasted lambs. Set aside for 10 minutes. Slice into chops.

Nutrition:

Calories:1750;

Carbohydrates: 15g;

Protein: 33g;

Fat: 20g;

Sugar: 2.2g;

Sodium: 579mg; Fiber: 1g

89. Pistachio-crusted Rack of Lamb

Preparation Time: 25 minutes

Cooking Time: 1 hour

Servings: 4

Ingredients

1 cup pomegranate juice

1/4 cup dried currants

1 garlic clove, peeled

3 tbsps. chilled butter, cut into 1/2-inch cubes

1/2 tsp. ground cinnamon

1/4 tsp. ground cumin

1 large rack of lamb (2 1/4 lbs.), well trimmed

1/4 cup chopped natural unsalted pistachios

1/4 cup panko (Japanese breadcrumbs)*

Direction

Preheat an oven to 400°F. Boil garlic, currants and pomegranate juice for 10 minutes till reduced to 1/4 cup and liquid is syrupy in medium skillet, mixing often.

Put mixture in mini processor. Add cumin, cinnamon and butter; blend till coarse puree foams. Put processor bowl in freeze to slightly firm butter for 10 minutes.

Line foil on small rimmed baking sheet. Put lamb on sheet, bone side down; sprinkle pepper and salt. Spread over with pomegranate butter; sprinkle panko and pistachios, pressing to adhere.

Roast the rack of lamb for 30 minutes till inserted instant-read thermometer into side reads 135°F for medium rare. Put on work surface; rest for 10 minutes. Between bones, cut lamb; drizzle juices from foil.

90. Provencal Lamb With Mediterranean Vegetables

Preparation Time: 1hour 5 minutes

Cooking Time: 4hours 5 minutes

Servings: 4

Ingredients

2 tsps. coriander seeds

2 tsps. fennel seeds

2 tsps. dried thyme

1 tsp. salt

1/2 tsp. ground black pepper

1 tsp. olive oil

1 8-rib rack of lamb (about 1 1/2 lbs.), well trimmed

Mediterranean Vegetables

Direction

Grind initial 3 ingredients coarsely in a spice grinder/blender; put into small bowl. Stir in pepper and salt. Rub oil on lamb then spice mixture.

Put lamb on baking sheet; sit for 1 hour.

Preheat an oven to 425°F. Roast the lamb for 25 minutes till inserted thermometer in middle of meat reads 130°F for medium-rare.

Sit for 10 minutes. Between ribs, cut lamb to chops; on each plate, put 2 chops. Put Mediterranean veggies alongside.

Nutrition:

Calories:380;

Carbohydrates: 5g;

Protein: 29.4g;

Fat: 10g;

Sugar: 0g;

Sodium: 456mg;

Fiber: 1g

91. Rack Of Lamb

Preparation Time: 15 minutes

Cooking Time: 5 minutes

Servings: 4

Ingredients

1 rack of lamb (2 lb.)

1 cup A.1. Garlic & Herb Marinade

Direction Arrange lamb rack in a shallow dish, meat side down. Stream marinade over lamb. Allow lamb to marinate in the fridge, flipping every 1 1/2 hours. Turn oven to 375°F to preheat. Take lamb out of the marinade; dispose used marinade. Arrange meat in a shallow roasting pan.

Bake lamb in the preheated oven until its internal temperature reaches 160°F for 30 to 45 minutes. Take out of the oven; allow to stand, covered, for 15 minutes before serving.

Nutrition:

Calories:220;

Carbohydrates: 6g;

Protein: 28g;

Fat: g;

Sugar: 2.1g;

Sodium: 432mg;

Fiber: 2g

92. Rack Of Lamb And Cherry Tomatoes

Servings: 4

Cooking Time: 2hours 10 minutes

Preparation Time: 10 minutes

Preparation Time: 10 minutes

Cooking Time: 2hours 10 minutes

Servings: 4

Ingredients

1 2-lb. rack of lamb (about 8 ribs)

3 tbsps. olive oil, divided

3 tsps. chopped fresh rosemary, divided

2 12-oz. containers cherry tomatoes

Direction

Preheat an oven to 425°F. Rub 1 tbsp. oil on lamb; sprinkle 1 1/2 tsp. rosemary then pepper and salt.

Put on big rimmed baking sheet. In a big bowl, put tomatoes, 1 1/2 tsp. rosemary and 2 tbsp. oil. Sprinkle pepper and salt; toss to coat then scatter around lamb. Roast tomatoes and lamb for 30 minutes till inserted thermometer in thickest lamb part reads 135°F for medium rare. Allow to rest for 10 minutes. Between bones, cut lamb to individual chops; put onto platter with the tomatoes.

Nutrition:Calories:737;

Carbohydrates: 6.5g;

Protein: 26g; Fat: 27g;

Sugar: 2.2g; Sodium: 102mg;

Fiber: 1g

93. Rack Of Lamb With Figs

Preparation Time: 30 minutes

Cooking Time: 1hour 15 minutes

Servings: 8

Ingredients

2 racks of lamb (2 lbs. each)

1 tsp. salt, divided

1 cup water

1 small onion, finely chopped

1 tbsp. canola oil

1 garlic clove, minced

2 tbsps. cornstarch

1 cup port wine or 1/2 cup grape juice plus 1/2 cup reduced-sodium beef broth

10 dried figs, halved

1/4 tsp. pepper

1/2 cup coarsely chopped walnuts, toasted

Direction

Use 1/2 tsp. of salt to rub lamb. On a rack set in a roasting pan coated with grease, arrange lamb with meat side facing up.

Bake at 375 degrees without a cover until reaching desired doneness (for medium-rare, a thermometer should register 145 degrees; medium, 160 degrees and well-done, 170 degrees), about 45 to 60 minutes.

Transfer to a serving platter and use foil to cover loosely. Put 1 cup of water into the roasting pan, then stir to loosen any browned bits from pan. Strain the mixture with a fine sieve, then put drippings aside.

Sauté onion in a small saucepan with oil until soft. Put in garlic and cook for 1 minute more. Stir in cornstarch until combined, then put in leftover salt, pepper, figs, drippings and wine gradually. Bring the mixture to a boil. Lower heat to moderately low and cook without a cover for 10 minutes, until sauce is thickened and figs are soft, while stirring sometimes.

Sprinkle walnuts over lamand serve together with fig sauce.

Nutrition:

Calories:364;

Carbohydrates: 6.5g;

Protein: 23g;

Fat: 16g;

Sugar: 2.2g;

Sodium: 254mg;

Fiber: 3g

94. Rack Of Lamb With Fresh Herbs

Preparation Time: 15 minutes

Cooking Time: 45 minutes

Servings: 4

Ingredients

1 tbsp. coarsely chopped fresh parsley or 1 tsp. dried parsley flakes

1 tbsp. olive oil

2 garlic cloves, minced

1 tsp. minced fresh rosemary or 1/4 tsp. dried rosemary, crushed

1 tsp. minced fresh thyme or 1/4 tsp. dried thyme

1/4 tsp. salt

1/4 tsp. Montreal steak seasoning

1/4 tsp. pepper

2 frenched racks of lamb (1-1/2 lbs. each)

1/4 cup pomegranate seeds

Direction

Set the oven to 375° and start preheating. Mix the first 8 ingredients in a small bowl. On a rack in a shallow roasting pan, put lamb; and rub the lamb with herb mixture.

Bake until meat reaches the doneness as desired, about 30-40 minutes (for those who like well-done meat, a thermometer should read 170°; for medium, 160°; for medium-rare, 145°).

Allow to sit 5 minutes before cutting. Serve with pomegranate seeds.

Nutrition:

Calories:865;

Carbohydrates: 4.5g;

Protein: 9g;

Fat: 3g;

Sugar: 2.1g;

Sodium: 564mg;

Fiber: 0g

95. Lamb With Pecan-chipotle Sauce

Preparation Time: 15 minutes

Cooking Time: 20 minutes

Servings: 4

Ingredients 2 tbsps. olive oil

1/2 small white onion, chopped

1 garlic clove, chopped

1/2 cup chopped pecans

4 cups water

8 fresh cilantro sprigs

1 tsp. finely chopped canned chipotle chiles plus 2 tbsps. adobo sauce

1/4 cup chile seeds (from any dried but not smoked chile, such as ancho or pasilla)

3/4 tsp. aniseed

1/2 tsp. ground allspice

1 (1-inch piece) canela* or cinnamon stick

2 whole cloves

2 (1 1/4- to 1 1/2-lb.) racks of lamb, fat trimmed, frenched (trimmed between bones)

Direction: In medium saucepan, heat oil over medium-high heat. Put in onion, sauté for 2 minutes or until translucent. Put in garlic, sauté for 1 minute.

Put in cilantro, pecans and 4 cups water. Boil for 10 minutes. Mix in adobo sauce and chipotle chiles. Take the cilantro out. In blender, puree the mixture. Put back to the saucepan, boil for 20 minutes or until reduced to one and a half cups. Season salt to the sauce.

Start preheating the oven to 350°F. In large skillet, toast chile seeds for 3 minutes over medium-high heat, until aromatic, shaking the pan constantly. Place the seeds into spice grinder. Put in spices and grind very finely. Sprinkle salt over the lamb.

Add spice mixture to coat. Arrange the lamb on the heavy rimmed baking sheet, bone side down. Roast lamb on medium-rare for 25 minutes or until thermometer reads 125°F when inserted into the thickest part of the meat.

Allow the lamb to stand for 5 minutes. Chop the lamb. Add the sauce over top and enjoy.

Nutrition: Calories:1015; Carbohydrates: 6.5g; Protein: 29g; Fat: 12g; Sugar: 0g; Sodium: 354mg; Fiber: 1.7g

96. Keto Rack Of Lamb With Port And Black Olive Sauce

Preparation Time: 15 minutes

Cooking Time: 1hour 15 minutes

Servings: 4

Ingredients

2 cups beef stock or canned beef broth

2 cups chicken stock or canned low-salt chicken broth

2/3 cup ruby Port

1/3 cup minced shallots

2 tsps. minced fresh thyme

2 tbsps. (1/4 stick) unsalted butter, room temperature

1 tbsp. all purpose flour

2 1 1/4- to 1 1/2-lb. racks of lamb, trimmed

1/4 cup Dijon mustard

3/4 cup (packed) fresh breadcrumbs from crustless French bread

3/4 cup freshly grated Parmesan cheese (about 2 1/4 oz.)

6 tbsps. chopped fresh parsley

3 tbsps. unsalted butter, melted

1 1/2 tbsps. minced garlic

1/2 cup chopped pitted Kalamata olives

Direction

Boil the first 5 ingredients for around 35 minutes in a large, heavy saucepan on medium-high heat, or till the mixture is reduced to 1 1/2 cups. In a small bowl, combine flour and 2 tbsps. of butter till a paste forms.

Whisk the paste into the sauce; simmer for around 3 minutes, or till thickened slightly. Strain into a heavy, small saucepan. Set the oven at 450°F and start preheating. Arrange lamb on a baking sheet. Spread with mustard.

In a small bowl, combine garlic, butter, parsley, cheese and breadcrumbs; press onto the lamb. Bake the lamb to the desired doneness, for around 25 minutes for medium-rare. Simmer the sauce.

Stir in olives. Cut the lamb between the ribs into chops. Serve accompanied with the sauce.

Nutrition:

Calories:1255;

Carbohydrates: 28g;

Protein: 49g;

Fat: 35g;

Sugar: 2.2g;

Sodium: 1215mg;

Fiber: 0.2g

97. Rack Of Lamb With Swiss Chard

Preparation Time: 1hour

Cooking Time: 4hours

Servings: 8

Ingredients

1/2 cup sweet (red) vermouth

1/2 cup golden raisins

1 medium onion, chopped

2 tbsps. extra-virgin olive oil

2 large bunches green Swiss chard (1 lb. total), stems and center ribs reserved for another use and leaves coarsely chopped

2 tbsps. pine nuts, toasted

4 (8-rib) frenched racks of lamb (each about 1 1/2 lb.), trimmed of all but a thin layer of fat

1/2 cup Dijon mustard

2 tsps. finely chopped thyme

1 tsp. finely chopped rosemary

Equipment: kitchen string

Accompaniment: roasted red peppers

Direction

Swiss chard stuffing: Boil raisins and vermouth in a small saucepan; take off heat. Steep for 15 minutes till raisins are plump and soft.

Cook onion in oil in a big heavy skillet on medium low heat for 5-8 minutes till onion is tender yet not brown, occasionally mixing. Add 1/4 tsp. pepper, 1/2 tsp. salt, raisins with any leftover vermouth and chard; cook on medium heat for 12 minutes till liquid evaporates and chard is tender, constantly turning chard with tongs. Put in a bowl; mix nuts in. Cool.

Lamb: create 1 long incision, cutting as near to bones as possible, to separate meat of every rack from bones, don't cut all the way through, stop 1/2-in. from the bottom. Roll away meat from bones to make long opening; season inside with pepper and salt. Use stuffing to fill; roll back meat over the stuffing. Use string to tie the meat to bones between every 2 ribs.

Preheat an oven with rack in the center to 400°F.

Mix rosemary, thyme and mustard; spread on both sides of every rack.

Put lamb racks in a big heavy shallow baking pan; pair racks so they stand up with bones interlocking yet leave space between them at the base.

Roast lamb for 25-35 minutes till inserted instant-read thermometer in the middle of the meat without touching the bone reads 130°F to get medium-rare; stand for 15 minutes, loosely covered.

Cut every rack for 4 double chops; discard the string. Serve over roasted red peppers.

You can make stuffing 1 da ahead, covered, chilled.

Nutrition:

Calories:3122;

Carbohydrates: 5g;

Protein: 121g;

Fat: 123g;

Sugar: 0.2g;

Sodium: 640mg;

Fiber: 1g

98. Roast Rack Of Lamb With Herb Sauce

Preparation Time: 35 minutes

Cooking Time: 1hour 10 minutes

Servings: 4

Ingredients

1/4 cup minced fresh rosemary

1-1/2 tsps. coarsely ground pepper

1-1/2 tsps. salt

2 racks of lamb (1-1/2 lbs. each)

1 tbsp. olive oil

SAUCE:

3/4 cup fresh parsley leaves

2/3 cup fresh basil leaves

1/3 cup each fresh cilantro leaves, mint leaves, oregano leaves and thyme leaves

1/3 cup coarsely chopped fresh chives

1/3 cup chopped shallots

2 garlic cloves, crushed

3 tbsps. grated lemon peel

1/2 cup lemon juice

2 tbsps. Dijon mustard

3/4 tsp. salt

1/2 tsp. pepper

1/3 cup olive oil

Direction

Mix salt, pepper and rosemary; rub on lamb. Refrigerate for 8 hours or overnight, covered.

Preheat an oven to 375°. Put lamb, fat side up, into a shallow roasting pan; drizzle with oil.

Roast for 35-45 minutes till meat gets desired doneness (170°: well-done, 160°: medium, 145°: medium-rare on a thermometer).

Take off lamb from oven; use foil to tent. Let sit for 10 minutes then serve.

Meanwhile, pulse garlic, shallots and herbs till herbs are chopped in a food processor.

Add pepper, salt, mustard, lemon juice and lemon peel; process till blended. In a steady stream, gradually add oil while processing; serve lamb with sauce.

Nutrition:

Calories:630;

Carbohydrates: 6.5g;

Protein: 4.2g;

Fat: 5g;

Sugar: 0.5g;

Sodium: 606mg;

Fiber: 0g

Squash Recipes.

99. Ham-stuffed Squash Boats

Preparation Time: 15 minutes

Cooking Time: 30 minutes

Servings: 4

Ingredients 1/4 tsp. pepper

4 medium yellow summer squash or zucchini (about 6 inches)

1 small onion, finely chopped

2 tbsps. butter

1 cup cubed fully cooked ham

1/2 cup dry bread crumbs

1/2 cup shredded cheddar cheese - 1/2 cup shredded Parmesan cheese, divided

1 egg, beaten 1 tsp. paprika

Direction

Cut squash lengthwise in half; scoop out pulp, keeping a 3/8-in. shell. Chop the pulp; set aside. Cook the shells for 4-5 minutes in a large saucepan of boiling water. Strain; set aside. Sauté onion in another saucepan with butter till tender; take away from the heat. Put in the squash pulp, pepper, paprika, egg, 1/4 cup of Parmesan cheese, Cheddar cheese, bread crumbs and ham. Combine thoroughly. Transfer into the shells with a spoon. Arrange on a baking sheet lightly coated with grease. Sprinkle the remaining Parmesan cheese over. Bake at 425° till heated through, or for 12-15 minutes.

Nutrition: Calories:318;
Carbohydrates: 6.5g;
Protein: 29.4g; Fat: 18g;
Sugar: 2g; Sodium: 897mg;
Fiber: 0g

100. Stuffed Yellow Summer Squash

Preparation Time: 20 minutes

Cooking Time: 1hour 25 minutes

Servings: 6

Ingredients: 3 cups water

1 (6 oz.) package wild rice

6 yellow squash, halved lengthwise

1 splash olive oil, or to taste

2 small summer squash, diced

2 bell peppers, or more to taste, diced

2 cucumbers, diced

1 onion, diced

3 cherry or grape tomatoes, or more to taste

1 cup shredded Gouda cheese

Direction: Boil wild rice and water in saucepan. Lower heat to medium low and cover; simmer for 30-45 minutes till rice is tender. Drain extra liquid; use fork to fluff rice. Cook for 5 more minutes, uncovered.

Preheat an oven to 175°C/350°F.

Put yellow squash halves on baking sheet.

In preheated oven, bake yellow squash for 20 minutes till tender.

In big skillet, heat olive oil on medium high heat; sauté tomatoes, onion, cucumbers, bell peppers and summer squash in hot oil for 5 minutes till tender.

Mound rice above each squash halve; put portion of sautéed veggie mixture on rice.

Put squash in preheated oven; bake for 30 more minutes.

Sprinkle gouda cheese on stuffed squash halves; bake for 5 minutes till cheese melts.

Nutrition: Calories:220; Fat: 5g; Carbohydrates: 16g; Fiber: 0g Protein: 32g; Sugar: 0.6g; Sodium: 544mg;

101. Chorizo Stuffed Squash

Preparation Time: 15 minutes

Cooking Time: 1 hour

Servings: 4

Ingredients

1 large pattypan squash, halved and seeded

1 cup water

1/2 (1 lb.) chorizo sausage

1 tbsp. olive oil

1 cup chopped onion

1 clove garlic, minced

1/2 green bell pepper, chopped

1 large tomato, chopped

1 cup chicken stock

1 cup black beans

1/2 cup corn

1 oz. shredded Cheddar cheese

Direction

Set the oven at 350°F (175°C) and start preheating. Place squash in a baking dish, cut-side down; put in water.

Bake in the preheated oven for around 30 minutes, till the squash becomes tender.

Place a large skillet on medium-high heat. Cook while stirring chorizo for 5-7 minutes in the hot skillet, till crumbly and browned; strain and discard the grease.

Place a separate skillet on medium heat; heat olive oil; cook while stirring garlic and onion for 10-15 minutes, till the onion is browned and softened. Put in green bell pepper; cook for 3-4 minutes, till softened. Put in corn, black beans, chicken stock and tomato; cook while stirring for around 10 minutes, till the liquid is evaporated. Mix in the chorizo. Turn the squash over; fill the chorizo mixture into each half; add Cheddar cheese on top.

Bake in the preheated oven for around 5 minutes, till the cheese is melted.

Nutrition:

Calories:532;

Carbohydrates: 15g;

Protein: 38g;

Fat: 6g;

Sugar: 0g;

Sodium: 997mg;

Fiber: 1.7g

102.   Squash And Zucchini Casserole

Preparation Time: 20 minutes

Cooking Time: 50 minutes

Servings: 5

Ingredients

2 medium yellow squash

2 large zucchini

1 Vidalia onions, thinly sliced

2 large tomatoes, sliced

2 cups grated Romano cheese

1/2 cup butter, divided

salt and pepper to taste

Direction

Start preheating the oven to 375°F (190°C).

Slice the squash and zucchini into long, thin layers. Lightly oil a 7x11-inch baking dish and arrange tomatoes, onion, zucchini, and squash in layer onto the baking dish. Spread with cheese and include in pats of butter between each layer of vegetables, and flavor each layer to taste with ground black pepper and salt.

Keep layering process until every vegetable are used and top with leftover cheese and butter. Bake, with cover, for 20 to 30 minutes at 375°F (190°C), until vegetables reach the desired tenderness and cheese melts and bubbles.

Nutrition:Calories:407;

Carbohydrates: 12;

Protein: 29.4g; Fat: 4.2g;

Sugar: 2.2g; Sodium: 721mg;

Fiber: 3g

103. Butternut Squash And Carrot Soup

Preparation Time: 15 minutes

Cooking Time: 50 minutes

Servings: 6

Ingredients

1 tbsp. butter or margarine

3 cups peeled, diced butternut squash (about 1 small squash)

2 cups thinly sliced carrots (4 medium carrots)

¾ cup thinly sliced leeks or chopped onion

2 (14.5 oz.) cans reduced-sodium chicken broth

¼ tsp. ground white pepper

¼ tsp. nutmeg

¼ cup regular or fat-free half-and-half or light cream

Fresh tarragon leaves (optional)

Direction

Melt the margarine or butter in a big saucepan on medium heat. Put onion or leeks, carrots and squash into the pan. Cook for 8 minutes, stirring once in a while, with cover. Put in broth then boil. Turn down the heat and let it simmer for 25 minutes, covered, or until the veggies become very soft.

In a blender container or food processor bowl, put 1/3 of the squash mixture. Put a cover and blend or process until it becomes nearly smooth. Redo the steps with the leftover mixture. Put the mixture back in the pan. Put in nutmeg and white pepper. Bring it just to a boil then add light cream or half-and-half; heat through. Scoop it into the bowls and if preferred, put fresh tarragon on top as garnish.

Nutrition:Calories:908;

Carbohydrates: 6.5g;

Protein: 36g; Fat: 8g;

Sugar: 0.3g; Sodium: 454mg;

Fiber: 1g

104. Curried Cheesy Cauliflower-squash Soup

Preparation Time: 20 minutes

Cooking Time: 45 minutes

Servings: 6

Ingredients

1 tbsp. olive oil

1 small onion, diced

2 cloves garlic, minced

4 cups chicken broth

1 head cauliflower, chopped

1 butternut squash, peeled and chopped

2 tbsps. yellow curry powder

1 tsp. salt, or to taste

3 cups shredded mozzarella and Cheddar cheese blend

Direction

Switch on a multi-functional pressure cooker (such as Instant Pot®), select the Sauté function, and allow to heat. Toss in olive oil and onion; sauté for about 3 minutes, until soft. Introduce garlic and sauté for another minute.

Mix in cauliflower, butternut squash and broth. Lock the lid; set vent to seal. According to manufacturer's instructions, select high pressure; put timer for 6 minutes. Allow pressure to build for 10 to 15 minutes.

Use the quick-release method according to the manufacturer's instructions to release pressure for about 5 minutes. Unlock the lid and remove it.

Stir salt and curry powder into the soup in the pressure cooker. Use an immersion blender to grind soup to desired texture.

Add Cheddar cheese blend and shredded mozzarella; immediately serve.

Nutrition: Calories:326;

Carbohydrates: 6g;

Protein: 29.4g; Fat: 17.3g;

Sugar: 4g; Sodium: 1514mg;

Fiber: 1.7g

105. Garlic-feta Roasted Butternut Squash With Chicken

Preparation Time: 15 minutes

Cooking Time: 45 minutes

Servings: 4

Ingredients

2 lbs. cubed butternut squash

2 large skinless, boneless chicken breasts, thinly sliced

1 large sweet red onion, or to taste, finely chopped

1 cup Mediterranean-style (with basil, Kalamata olive, and sun-dried tomato) crumbled feta cheese

2 tbsps. extra-virgin olive oil

2 cloves garlic, or to taste, minced

1 pinch ground multi-colored peppercorns, or to taste

1 pinch sea salt, or to taste

Direction

Preheat oven to 400 °F (200 °C).

In a roasting pan, mix chicken, olive oil, butternut squash, garlic, feta cheese, red onion, sea salt and pepper together.

In preheated oven, roast for around 30 to 40 minutes (for every ten minutes or so, stirring) until the squash cubes are soft and the chicken is no longer pink in the center.

Nutrition:

Calories:405;

Carbohydrates: 21g;

Protein: 34.4g;

Fat: 5g;

Sugar: 0g;

Sodium: 583mg;

Fiber: 1.7g

106. Chicken Paprika With Spaghetti Squash

Preparation Time: 30 minutes

Cooking Time: 2 hours

Servings: 66

Ingredients

1 (3 lb.) spaghetti squash

2 tbsps. olive oil

1 onion, thinly sliced

2 cloves garlic, minced

1 green bell pepper, diced

2 tbsps. paprika

1 tsp. salt

1 tsp. caraway seeds

ground black pepper to taste

3 skinless, boneless chicken breast halves

1 (14.5 oz.) can whole peeled tomatoes, drained

1/2 cup sour cream (optional)

Direction

Preheat the oven to 175 °C or 350 °F. Prick squash in few areas with a fork or skewer. On a baking sheet, put the uncut squash; let roast for 45 minutes. Flip the squash over and allow to roast for 10 minutes more. Reserve to cool.

In a big skillet over moderate-high heat, heat the olive oil. In hot oil, cook and mix ground black pepper, caraway seeds, salt, paprika, green bell pepper, garlic and onion for 5 minutes till onion is translucent and tender.

Take off from skillet and reserve, retaining olive oil in the pan.

Turn heat to medium and allow chicken breasts to cook for 10 minutes each side using the same skillet till meat is not pink on the inside anymore, juices run clear and browned, flipping one time. Take off chicken breasts and cut diagonally. Put onion mixture and chicken back to pan; mix in the tomatoes. Simmer chicken mixture.

Halve the squash and using a spoon, scrape out seeds. Pull out squash strands from peels with a fork. With vegetables and chicken, mix the squash, raise heat, and boil. Turn heat to low and allow to simmer for 10 minutes to incorporate flavors. Mix in sour cream if wished

Nutrition:

Calories:308;

Carbohydrates: 8g;

Protein: 15.4g;

Fat: 11g;

Sugar: 2.2g;

Sodium: 561mg;

Fiber: 0.3g

107. Chicken, Arugula & Butternut Squash Salad With Brussels Sprouts

Preparation Time: 15 minutes

Cooking Time: 35 minutes

Servings: 4

Ingredients

2¾ cups precubed butternut squash

2½ cups halved Brussels sprouts (or quartered, if large)

1 tsp. extra-virgin olive oil

¾ tsp. salt, divided

⅛ tsp. ground pepper plus ¼ tsp., divided

2 cups cubed cooked chicken (½-inch; about 10 oz.)

1 cup red grapes, halved

½ cup very thinly sliced red onion

1 5-oz. package baby arugula

¼ cup walnut oil or extra-virgin olive oil

2 tbsps. white-wine vinegar

2 tbsps. finely chopped shallot

2 tsps. Dijon mustard

Direction

Preheat oven to 425 °F. In a large rimmed baking sheet, use cooking spray to coat.

In a large bowl, toss 1/8 tsp. pepper, 1 tsp. olive oil, Brussels sprouts, 1/4 tsp. salt and squash. On the prepared baking sheet, place in a single layer (reserve the bowl). Roast for around 20 to 22 minutes, stirring once or twice, until the vegetables are soft.

In the reserved bowl, combine grapes, chicken, arugula and onion. Put in the roasted vegetables and combine by tossing.

In a small bowl, whisk vinegar, walnut oil (or olive oil), the rest of 1/2 tsp. salt, mustard, shallot and 1/4 tsp. pepper.

Pour over the salad and toss gently for combining.

Nutrition:

Calories:240;

Carbohydrates: 10g;

Protein: 17g;

Fat: 6g;

Sugar: 7g;

Sodium: 378mg;

Fiber: 3g

108. Couscous-stuffed Acorn Squash

Preparation Time: 15 minutes

Cooking Time: 1hour 3 minutes

Servings: 2

Ingredients

1 acorn squash, halved and seeded

2 1/4 cups water

1 1/2 cups whole wheat couscous

2 tbsps. chopped fresh cilantro

1 bunch fresh spinach, trimmed and coarsely chopped

1 tbsp. margarine

1/2 small onion, chopped

1/2 tsp. seasoned salt, or to taste (optional)

salt and ground black pepper to taste

1/4 cup crumbled feta cheese

Direction

Set the oven to 350°F (175°C) for preheating. In a baking sheet, arrange the acorn squash cut-side down.

Bake the squash inside the preheated oven for 45 minutes until the squash is tender when pierced using the fork. Flip the squash up and allow it to cool slightly.

Boil 2 1/4 cups of water in a saucepan. Remove it from the heat and mix in cilantro and couscous. Cover the saucepan. Allow it to stand for 10 minutes until the water is completely absorbed. Use a fork to fluff the couscous.

Boil a large pot of water. Add the spinach and let it cook for 3-5 minutes until wilted. Drain and use a paper towel to squeeze out any remaining moisture. Fold it into the couscous.

In a skillet, melt the margarine. Add the onion and cook and stir for 10 minutes until browned. Stir onion into the couscous mixture. Mix in salt, pepper, and seasoned salt.

Along with the couscous mixture, stuff the acorn squash halves. Top the acorn squash with feta cheese.

Let it bake inside the preheated oven for 15 minutes until heated through.

Nutrition:

Calories:908;

Carbohydrates: 3.4g;

Protein: 35g;

Fat: 8g;

Sugar: 2g;

Sodium: 877mg;

Fiber: 1.7g

109. Pork With Squash

Preparation Time: 10 minutes

Cooking Time: 2hours 28 minutes

Servings: 8

Ingredients

2 tbsps. olive oil, divided

4 boneless pork chops

5 calabaza squash, halved and sliced 1/2-inch thick

1 cup whole kernel corn, drained

1/2 cup chopped onion

1/2 cup chopped tomatoes

2 tsps. minced garlic

1 (6 oz.) can tomato sauce

1/2 tsp. ground cumin

1/4 tsp. salt

1/4 tsp. ground black pepper

1/4 tsp. garlic powder

2 cups chicken stock, or more as needed

Direction

Heat 1 tbsp. of olive oil on medium-high heat in a saucepan. Cook pork chops about 4 minutes each side until not pink anymore in the center. Let cool about 5 minutes until easy to handle. Slice the pork into bite-sized cubes.

In the saucepan, heat 1 tbsp. leftover olive oil. Include in garlic, tomatoes, onion, corn, Calabaza squash, and cubed pork; cook about 5 minutes until onion is translucent. Blend in garlic powder, pepper, salt, cumin, and tomato sauce.

Put in chicken stock; cover and simmer about 2 hours until flavors combine.

Stir from time to time and monitor periodically to check if additional chicken stock if necessary.

Nutrition: Calories:348;

Carbohydrates: 6.5g;

Protein: 15.4g; Fat: 8g;

Sugar: 2.2g; Sodium: 477mg;

Fiber: 1.7g

110. Easy Slow Cooker Butternut Squash Soup

Preparation Time: 20 minutes

Cooking Time: 8hours 30 minutes

Servings: 4

Ingredients: 1 tbsp. olive oil

2 onions, chopped

2 tsps. dried rosemary

1/2 tsp. ground black pepper

5 cups vegetable stock

1 butternut squash - peeled, seeded, and cut into cubes

2 Granny Smith apples - peeled, cored, and chopped

salt to taste

1 cup shredded Swiss cheese

1/2 cup finely chopped walnuts

Direction

In a big frying pan, heat oil over medium heat. Stir and cook onions in the hot oil for 5-10 minutes until tender. Mix in black pepper and rosemary, move the mixture to a slow cooker. Add apples, butternut squash, and vegetable stock to the slow cooker.

Cook for 8 hours on Low (or 4 hours on high).

Put the oven rack approximately 6-inch from the heat source and start preheating the oven's broiler.

With an immersion blender, puree the soup until smooth. Or you can add the soup to a food processor and puree in batches until smooth. Use salt to season.

Pour the soup into oven-safe bowls and sprinkle over the top with walnuts and Swiss cheese.

Cook the soup under the preheated broiler for 1-2 minutes until the cheese is bubbly and hot.

Nutrition: Calories:206;

Carbohydrates: 15g;

Protein: 33g; Fat: 12g;

Sugar: 6g; Sodium: 223 mg;

Fiber: 0g

111. Cheesy Summer Squash Flatbreads

Preparation Time: 15 minutes

Cooking Time: 30 minutes

Servings: 4

Ingredients

3 small yellow summer squash, sliced 1/4 inch thick

1 tbsp. olive oil

1/2 tsp. salt

2 cups fresh baby spinach, coarsely chopped

2 naan flatbreads

1/3 cup roasted red pepper hummus

1 carton (8 oz.) fresh mozzarella cheese pearls

Pepper

Direction

Heat the oven to 425 degrees. Toss squash with salt and oil; scatter evenly in a 15x10x1-inch baking pan. Roast for 8 to 10 minutes or until tender. Place to a bowl; mix in spinach.

Put naan on a baking sheet; smear hummus on.

Place cheese and squash mixture on top. Put on a lower oven rack and bake for 4-6 minutes or just until cheese melts.

Dust with pepper.

Nutrition

Calories: 332 calories

Total Carbohydrate: 24 g

Cholesterol: 47 mg

Total Fat: 20 g

Fiber: 3 g

Protein: 15 g

Sodium: 737 mg

Soup Recipes

112. Cream Zucchini Soup

Preparation Time: 8-10 minutes

Cooking Time: 8 minutes

Servings: 4

Ingredients:

2 cups vegetable stock

2 garlic cloves, crushed

1 tablespoon butter

4 (preferably medium size) zucchinis, peeled and chopped

1 small onion, chopped

2 cups heavy cream

1/2 teaspoon dried oregano, (finely ground)

1/2 teaspoon black pepper, (finely ground)

1 teaspoon dried parsley, (finely ground)

1 teaspoon of sea salt

Lemon juice (optional)

Directions:

Arrange Instant Pot over a dry platform in your kitchen. Open its top lid and switch it on.

Find and press "SAUTE" cooking function; add the butter in it and allow it to melt.

In the pot, add the onions, zucchini, garlic; cook (while stirring) until turns translucent and softened for around 2-3 minutes.

Add the vegetable broth and sprinkle with salt, oregano, pepper, and parsley; gently stir to mix well.

Close the lid to create a locked chamber; make sure that safety valve is in locking position.

Find and press "MANUAL" cooking function; timer to 5 minutes with default "HIGH" pressure mode.

Allow the pressure to build to cook the ingredients.

After cooking time is over press "CANCEL" setting. Find and press "QPR" cooking function. This setting is for quick release of inside pressure.

Slowly open the lid, take out the cooked recipe in serving plates or serving bowls, and enjoy the keto recipe. Top with some lemon juice.

Nutrition:

Calories:490;

Carbohydrates: 11g;

Protein: 23g;

Fat: 6g;

Sugar: 2.2g;

Sodium: 564mg;

Fiber: 1.7g

113. Coconut Chicken Soup

Preparation Time: 10 minutes

Cooking Time: 18 minutes

Servings: 4

Ingredients:

4 cloves of garlic, minced

1 pound chicken breasts, skin-on

4 cups of water

2 tablespoons olive oil

1 onion, diced

1 cup of coconut milk

(finely ground) black pepper and salt as per taste preference

2 tablespoons sesame oil

Directions:

Arrange Instant Pot over a dry platform in your kitchen. Open its top lid and switch it on.

Find and press "SAUTE" cooking function; add the oil in it and allow it to heat.

In the pot, add the onions, garlic; cook (while stirring) until turns translucent and softened for around 1-2 minutes.

Stir in the chicken breasts; stir, and cook for 2 more minutes.

Pour in water and coconut milk — season to taste.

Close the lid to create a locked chamber; make sure that safety valve is in locking position.

Find and press "MANUAL" cooking function; timer to 15 minutes with default "HIGH" pressure mode.

Allow the pressure to build to cook the ingredients.

After cooking time is over press "CANCEL" setting. Find and press "NPR" cooking function. This setting is for the natural release of inside pressure and it takes around 10 minutes to slowly release pressure.

Slowly open the lid, Drizzle with sesame oil on top.

Take out the cooked recipe in serving plates or serving bowls and enjoy the keto recipe.

Nutrition:

Calories:328;

Carbohydrates: 6g;

Protein: 21g;

Fat: 0g;

Sugar: 6g;

Sodium: 609mg;

Fiber: 2g

114.   Chicken Bacon Soup

Preparation Time: 10 minutes

Cooking Time: 40 minutes

Servings: 4

Ingredients:

6 boneless, skinless chicken thighs, make cubes

½ cup chopped celery

4 minced garlic cloves

6-ounce mushrooms, sliced

½ cup chopped onion

8-ounce softened cream cheese

¼ cup softened butter

1 teaspoon dried thyme

Salt and (finely ground) black pepper, as per taste preference

2 cups chopped spinach

8 ounces cooked bacon slices, chopped

3 cups (preferably homemade) chicken broth

1 cup heavy cream

Directions:

Arrange Instant Pot over a dry platform in your kitchen. Open its top lid and switch it on.

Add the ingredients except for the cream, spinach, and bacon; gently stir to mix well.

Close the lid to create a locked chamber; make sure that safety valve is in locking position.

Find and press "SOUP" cooking function; timer to 30 minutes with default "HIGH" pressure mode.

Allow the pressure to build to cook the ingredients.

After cooking time is over press "CANCEL" setting. Find and press "NPR" cooking function. This setting is for the natural release of inside pressure and it takes around 10 minutes to slowly release pressure.

Slowly open the lid, stir in cream and spinach.

Take out the cooked recipe in serving plates or serving bowls and enjoy the keto recipe. Top with the bacon.

Nutrition:

Calories:490;

Carbohydrates: 7g;

Protein: 23g;

Fat: 6g;

Sugar: 2.2g;

Sodium: 742mg;

Fiber: 1.7g

115. Cream Pepper Soup

Preparation Time: 8-10 minutes

Cooking Time: 10 minutes

Servings: 4

Ingredients:

1 (preferably medium size) celery stalk, chopped

1 (preferably medium size) yellow bell pepper, chopped

1 (preferably medium size) green bell pepper, chopped

2 large red bell peppers, chopped

1 small red onion, chopped

2 tablespoons butter

1/2 cup cream cheese, full-fat

1/4 teaspoon dried thyme, (finely ground)

1/2 teaspoon black pepper, (finely ground)

1 teaspoon dried parsley, (finely ground)

1 teaspoon salt

2 cups vegetable stock

1 cup heavy cream

Directions:

Arrange Instant Pot over a dry platform in your kitchen. Open its top lid and switch it on.

Find and press "SAUTE" cooking function; add the butter in it and allow it to heat. In the pot, add the onions, bell pepper, and celery; cook (while stirring) until turns translucent and softened for around 3-4 minutes.

Pour in the vegetable stock and heavy cream — season with salt, pepper, parsley, and thyme.

Close the lid to create a locked chamber; make sure that safety valve is in locking position.

Find and press "MANUAL" cooking function; timer to 6 minutes with default "HIGH" pressure mode.

Allow the pressure to build to cook the ingredients.

After cooking time is over press "CANCEL" setting. Find and press "QPR" cooking function. This setting is for quick release of inside pressure.

Slowly open the lid, mix in the cream; take out the cooked recipe in serving plates or serving bowls, and enjoy the keto recipe.

Nutrition:

Calories:286;

Carbohydrates: 9g;

Protein: 4g;

Fat: 0g;

Sugar: 2g;

Sodium: 445mg;

Fiber: 0g

116.   Ham Asparagus Soup

Preparation Time: 10 minutes

Cooking Time: 55 minutes

Servings: 4

Ingredients:

5 crushed garlic cloves

1 cup chopped ham

4 cups (preferably homemade) chicken broth

2 pounds trimmed and halved asparagus spears

2 tablespoons butter

1 chopped yellow onion

½ teaspoon dried thyme

Salt and freshly (finely ground) black pepper, as per taste preference

Directions:

Arrange Instant Pot over a dry platform in your kitchen. Open its top lid and switch it on.

Find and press "SAUTE" cooking function; add the butter in it and allow it to heat.

In the pot, add the onions; cook (while stirring) until turns translucent and softened for around 4-5 minutes.

Add the garlic, ham bone and broth; stir, and cook for about 2-3 minutes.

Add the other ingredients; gently stir to mix well.

Close the lid to create a locked chamber; make sure that safety valve is in locking position.

Find and press "SOUP" cooking function; timer to 45 minutes with default "HIGH" pressure mode.

Allow the pressure to build to cook the ingredients.

After cooking time is over press "CANCEL" setting. Find and press "QPR" cooking function. This setting is for quick release of inside pressure.

Slowly open the lid, add the prepared recipe mix in a blender or processor.

Blend or process to make a smooth mix. Place the mix in serving bowls and enjoy the keto recipe.

Nutrition:Calories:146;

Carbohydrates: 5g;

Protein: 29.4g;

Fat: 6g;

Sugar: 2.2g;

Sodium: 222mg;

Fiber: 4g

117.   Beef Zoodle Soup

Preparation Time: 5 minutes

Cooking Time: 13 minutes

Servings: 4

Ingredients:

Avocado oil – 4 tablespoons

Minced ginger – 3 tablespoons

Minced garlic – 1 tablespoon

Sirloin steak tips, cut into 1-inch pieces – 1 ½ pound

Broccoli florets – 2 cups

Bella mushrooms, sliced – 8 ounces

Beef broth – 6 cups

Apple cider vinegar – 1/4 cup

Coconut aminos – 1/4 cup

Sriracha sauce – 1/4 cup

large zucchini, spiralized into noodles – 1

Directions:

Switch on the instant pot, grease pot with oil, press the 'sauté/simmer' button, wait until the oil is hot and add the steak pieces along with ginger and garlic.

Cook steak for 5 minutes or more until nicely golden brown, then add remaining ingredients except for zucchini and stir until mixed.

Press the 'keep warm' button, shut the instant pot with its lid in the sealed position, then press the 'manual' button, press '+/-' to set the cooking time to 8 minutes and cook at high-pressure setting; when the pressure builds in the pot, the cooking timer will start.

When the instant pot buzzes, press the 'keep warm' button, do a quick pressure release and open the lid.

Taste the soup to adjust seasoning, add zucchini noodles and toss until just mixed.

Ladle the soup into bowls and serve.

Nutrition:

Calories:239;

Carbohydrates: 3g;

Protein: 29g;

Fat: 11g;

Sugar: 5g;

Sodium: 254mg;

Fiber: 1g

118. Broccoli Cheese Soup

Preparation Time: 10 minutes

Cooking Time: 12 minutes

Servings: 5

Ingredients:

Butter, unsalted – 2 tablespoons

Minced garlic – 2 tablespoons

Vegetable broth – 3 cups

Broccoli florets – 6-ounce

Monterey jack cheese, shredded – 1 cup

Sharp cheddar cheese, shredded – 2 cups, and 2 tablespoons

Dijon mustard – 1 tablespoon

Paprika – ½ teaspoon

Ground black pepper – ⅛ teaspoon

Heavy whipping cream – 1 cup

Salt – ¼ teaspoon

Xanthan gum – 1 teaspoon

Directions:

Switch on the instant pot, add butter, press the 'sauté/simmer' button, wait until the butter melts and add garlic and cook for 1 minute or until fragrant.

Stir in broth, cook for 1 minute, then add broccoli florets and stir until mixed.

Press the 'keep warm' button, shut the instant pot with its lid in the sealed position, then press the 'manual' button, press '+/-' to set the cooking time to 10 minutes and cook at high-pressure setting; when the pressure builds in the pot, the cooking timer will start.

When the instant pot buzzes, press the 'keep warm' button, do quick pressure release and open the lid.

Add mustard, Monterey jack cheese, and 2 cups of cheddar cheese, season with black pepper and paprika and stir until cheese begins to melt.

Then pour in the cream, stir until well-incorporated and taste to adjust salt.

Take out ¾ cup of soup, add xanthan gum, stir well, then add into the soup in the instant pot and stir well until well combined.

Garnish soup with remaining cheddar cheese and serve.

Nutrition:Calories:276;

Carbohydrates: 5.1g;

Protein: 11.8g; Fat: 23.8g;

Sugar: 2.2g; Sodium: 509mg;

Fiber: 0g

119.   Zuppa Toscana

Preparation Time: 10 minutes

Cooking Time: 25 minutes

Servings: 4

Ingredients:

Slices of bacon, chopped – 6

Ground Italian sausage – 1 pound

Butter, unsalted – 1 tablespoon

Minced garlic – 2 teaspoons

Ground sage – ½ teaspoon

Ground black pepper – ¼ teaspoon

Chicken broth – 2 ¾ cups

Heavy whipping cream – ¾ cup

Parmesan cheese, shredded – ¼ cup

Radishes, peeled, quartered – 1 pound

Kale, de-stemmed, leaves chopped – 2 ounces

Directions:

Switch on the instant pot, grease pot with oil, press the 'sauté/simmer' button, wait until the oil is hot, add sausage and cook for 5 minutes or until browned.

Transfer sausage to a plate, add bacon in the pot and cook for 4 minutes or until crispy.

Transfer bacon to a cutting board, let sit for 5 minutes and then chop it.

Add garlic in the instant pot, cook for 1 minute or until fragrant, then return sausage and bacon into the pot, add remaining ingredients except for cream, cheese, and kale and stir until mixed.

Press the 'keep warm' button, shut the instant pot with its lid in the sealed position, then press the 'manual' button, press '+/-' to set the cooking time to 10 minutes and cook at high-pressure setting; when the pressure builds in the pot, the cooking timer will start.

When the instant pot buzzes, press the 'keep warm' button, do a quick pressure release and open the lid.

Add remaining ingredients, stir well, press the 'sauté/simmer' button and simmer the soup for 5 minutes or until kale is tender. Ladle soup into bowls and serve.

Nutrition:

Calories:316;

Carbohydrates: 6.5g;

Protein: 13g;

Fat: 25g;

Sugar: 7g;

Sodium: 877mg;

Fiber: 1g

120. Thai Shrimp Soup

Preparation Time: 5 minutes

Cooking Time: 25 minutes

Servings: 6

Ingredients:

Butter, unsalted – 2 tablespoons

Medium shrimp, uncooked, peeled and deveined – ½ pound

White onion, peeled and diced – ½

Minced garlic – 1 tablespoon

Chicken broth – 4 cups

Lime juice – 2 tablespoons

Fish sauce – 2 tablespoons

Red curry paste – 2½ teaspoon

Coconut aminos – 1 tablespoon

Stalk of lemongrass, chopped – 1

Sliced fresh white mushrooms – 1 cup

Grated ginger – 1 tablespoon

Sea salt – 1 teaspoon

Ground black pepper – ½ teaspoon

Coconut milk, unsweetened, full-fat – 13.66-ounce

Chopped fresh cilantro – 3 tablespoons

Directions:

Switch on the instant pot, add 1 tablespoon butter, press the 'sauté/simmer' button, wait until butter melts, add shrimps, stir well and cook for 3 to 5 minutes or until shrimps turn pink.

Transfer shrimps to a plate, add remaining butter and when it melts, add onion and garlic and cook for 3 minutes.

Add remaining ingredients, reserving coconut milk, shrimps and cilantro, stir until mixed and press the 'keep warm' button.

Shut the instant pot with its lid in the sealed position, then press the 'manual' button, press '+/-' to set the cooking time to 5 minutes and cook at high-pressure setting; when the pressure builds in the pot, the cooking timer will start.

When the instant pot buzzes, press the 'keep warm' button, release pressure naturally for 5 minutes, then do a quick pressure release and open the lid.

Return shrimps into the instant pot, pour in milk, then press the 'sauté/simmer' button and bring the soup to boil.

Press the 'keep warm' button, let soup rest for 2 minutes and then ladle soup into bowls.

Garnish the soup with cilantro and serve.

Nutrition:

Calories:200;

Carbohydrates: 4g;

Protein: 15g;

Fat: 13g;

Sugar: 4

Sodium: 454mg;

Fiber: 0g

121. Chicken and Vegetable Soup

Preparation Time: 5 minutes

Cooking Time: 10 minutes

Servings: 4

Ingredients:

Butter, unsalted – 4 tablespoons

White onion, peeled and diced – 1/2 cup

Carrots, peeled and sliced – 1 cup

Stalks of celery, sliced – 2

Minced garlic – 1 ½ tablespoon

Chicken broth – 8 cups

Chicken thighs, skinless, boneless – 6

Fresh dill – 2 teaspoons

Fresh thyme – 2 teaspoons

Salt – 1 ½ teaspoon

Ground black pepper – 1 teaspoon

Avocado oil – 2 tablespoons

Directions:

Switch on the instant pot, add butter, press the 'sauté/simmer' button, wait until the oil is hot and add the onion, carrot, celery, and garlic and cook for 5 minutes or until sautéd.

Meanwhile, prepare the chicken and for this, cut chicken into bite-size pieces.

Add chicken into vegetables along with remaining ingredients, reserving the oil, and stir until just mixed.

Press the 'keep warm' button, shut the instant pot with its lid in the sealed position, then press the 'manual' button, press '+/-' to set the cooking time to 4 minutes and cook at high-pressure setting; when the pressure builds in the pot, the cooking timer will start.

When the instant pot buzzes, press the 'keep warm' button, release pressure naturally for 10 minutes, then do a quick pressure release and open the lid.

Ladle the soup into bowls, drizzle with oil and serve.

Nutrition:

Calories:330;

Carbohydrates: 6g;

Protein: 26g;

Fat: 21g;

Sugar: 2.2g;

Sodium: 254mg;

Fiber: 2g

122. Buffalo Ranch Chicken Dip

Preparation Time: 5 minutes

Cooking Time: 15 minutes

Servings: 4

Ingredients:

Chicken breast – 1 pound

Packet of ranch dip – 1

Hot sauce – 1 cup

Stick of butter, unsalted – 1

Cheddar cheese, grated – 16 ounces

Cream cheese – 8 ounces

Directions:

Switch on the instant pot and place all the ingredients except for cheddar cheese.

Shut the instant pot with its lid in the sealed position, then press the 'manual' button, press '+/-' to set the cooking time to 15 minutes and cook at high-pressure setting; when the pressure builds in the pot, the cooking timer will start.

When the instant pot buzzes, press the 'keep warm' button, do quick pressure release and open the lid.

Shred chicken with two forks, then add cheddar cheese and stir well until cheese completely melts.

Serve with vegetable sticks.

Nutrition:

Calories:526;

Carbohydrates: 2.5g;

Protein: 37g; Fat: 12g;

Sugar: 2.2g; Sodium: 254mg;

Fiber: 1.7g

123.   Creamy Taco Soup

Preparation Time: 5 minutes

Cooking Time: 10 minutes

Servings: 6

Ingredients:

Ground beef – 2 pounds

Minced garlic – 2 tablespoons

Red chili powder – 2 tablespoons

Cumin – 2 teaspoons

Diced tomatoes with chilies – 20 ounces

Beef broth – 32 ounces

Salt – 1 ½ teaspoon

Ground black pepper – ¾ teaspoon

Cream cheese – 8 ounces

Heavy cream – 1/2 cup

Directions:

Switch on the instant pot, press the 'sauté/simmer' button, wait until the pot is hot, then add ground beef and cook for 5 minutes or more until nicely browned.

Add remaining ingredients except for cream cheese, stir until mixed, then press the 'keep warm' button and shut the instant pot with its lid in the sealed position.

Press the 'soup' button, press '+/-' to set the cooking time to 5 minutes and cook at high-pressure setting; when the pressure builds in the pot, the cooking timer will start.

When the instant pot buzzes, press the 'keep warm' button, release pressure naturally for 10 minutes, then do a quick pressure release and open the lid.

Add cream cheese, stir well until combined and serve.

Nutrition:Calories:386;

Carbohydrates: 7g;

Protein: 27g;

Fat: 28g; Sugar: 2.2g;

Sodium: 254mg;

Fiber: 1g

124.   Chicken Kale Soup

Preparation Time: 10 minutes

Cooking Time: 25 minutes

Servings: 4

Ingredients:

Baby kale leaves – 5 ounces

Chicken breast, cubed – 2 pounds

Sliced white onion – 1/3 cup

Salt – 1 teaspoon

Avocado oil – ½ cup and 1 tablespoon

Chicken broth – 14 ounces

Chicken stock – 32 ounces

Lemon juice – 1/4 cup

Directions:

Switch on the instant pot, grease pot with 1 tablespoon oil, press the 'sauté/simmer' button, and wait until the oil is hot.

Sprinkle chicken with salt and black pepper until seasoned well, then add into the instant pot and cook for 3 to 5 minutes or until browned on all sides.

Press the 'keep warm' button, shut the instant pot with its lid in the sealed position and let it sit for 15 minutes or until the internal temperature of chicken reach to 165 degrees F.

Meanwhile, pour chicken broth in a blender, add onion and remaining oil and pulse until smooth.

Open the lid of the instant pot, shred chicken with two forks, pour in onion mixture along with remaining ingredients, stir well and shut with lid.

Press the 'manual' button, press '+/-' to set the cooking time to 10 minutes and cook at high-pressure setting; when the pressure builds in the pot, the cooking timer will start.

When the instant pot buzzes, press the 'keep warm' button, release pressure naturally for 10 minutes, then do a quick pressure release and open the lid.

Ladle soup into bowls and serve.

Nutrition:

Calories:261;

Carbohydrates: 1.2g;

Protein: 29.4g;

Fat: 21g;

Sugar: 3.2g;

Sodium: 258mg;

Fiber: 0.7g

125. Chicken Thigh Soup

Preparation Time: 5 minutes

Cooking Time: 30 minutes

Servings: 6

Ingredients:

Chicken thighs, with skin and bones – 2 pounds

Stalks of celery, chopped – 4

Radishes, peeled and chopped – 0.65 pounds

Small white onion, peeled and chopped – 1/2

Rosemary, chopped – 1 tablespoon

Basil, chopped – 1 tablespoon

Minced garlic – 1 tablespoon

Salt – 1/2 teaspoon

Ground black pepper – 1/4 teaspoon

Chicken broth – 4 cups

Bay leaves – 2

Directions:

Switch on the instant pot and place all the ingredients in it, with chicken thighs in the end.

Shut the instant pot with its lid in the sealed position, then press the 'soup' button, press '+/-' to set the cooking time to 30 minutes and cook at high-pressure setting; when the pressure builds in the pot, the cooking timer will start.

When the instant pot buzzes, press the 'keep warm' button, release pressure naturally and open the lid.

Transfer chicken thighs to a cutting board, separate its meat from th3 skin and bones, then cut the chicken into bite-sized pieces and return into the soup. Taste soup to adjust seasoning, then ladle into bowls and serve.

Nutrition:

Calories:356

Carbohydrates: 3g;

Protein: 25g;

Fat: 25g;

Sugar: 1g;

Sodium: 465mg;

Fiber: 4g

Snack Recipes.

126.   Apple Crisp

Preparation Time: 5 minutes

Cooking Time: 2 minutes

Servings: 6

Ingredients:

5 cups sliced apples

1 1/2 cups vanilla chia granola

1/2 teaspoon ground ginger

1/2 lemon, zested

1/4 cup brown sugar

1 1/8 teaspoon cinnamon

2 tablespoons maple syrup

1 teaspoon vanilla extract, unsweetened

1/4 cup coconut oil

2/3 cup water

Coconut whipped cream for serving

Directions:

Take a small bowl, add granola into it along with 2 tablespoons sugar and coconut oil and stir until well combined.

Switch on the instant pot, place apples in the inner pot, sprinkle with remaining sugar, ginger, and 1 teaspoon cinnamon, drizzle with maple and vanilla, pour in water, spread the apple slices in an even layer and cover evenly with granola mixture.

Shut the pot with the lid in the sealed position, press the manual button, press the +/- button to set the cooking time to 2 minutes, press the pressure level to select the high-pressure setting, and let cook; the instant pot will take 10 minutes to preheat and then the timer will start.

When it's done and the timer beeps, release the pressure through quick pressure release; this will take 3 minutes, and then carefully move the vent to "venting."

Meanwhile, take a small bowl, add lemon zest and remaining cinnamon and stir until mixed.

Open the instant pot, let the apple crisp stand for 5 minutes until the sauce has thickened, and distribute it into bowls.

Garnish apple crisp with lemon zest mixture and serve with coconut whipped cream.

Nutrition:

Calories:293;

Carbohydrates: 13.3g;

Protein: 4.5g;

Fat: 13.3g;

Sugar: 3g;

Sodium: 765mg;

Fiber: 2g

127.   Soy Milk Yogurt

Preparation Time: 5 minutes

Cooking Time: 14 hours

Servings: 4

Ingredients:

32 ounces of soy milk

2 tablespoons almond yogurt

Directions:

Take two-pint jars, divide soy milk into them evenly, then add 1 tablespoon of yogurt into each jar and stir until well mixed.

Switch on the instant pot, place the jars in the inner pot and shut the pot with the lid in the sealed position.

Press the yogurt button, press the +/- button to set the cooking time to 14 hours, press the pressure level to select the high-pressure setting, and let cook; the instant pot will take 10 minutes to preheat and then the timer will start.

When it's done and the timer beeps, move the vent to "venting," open the lid and take out the yogurt jars.

Stir in the yogurt and serve straight away or refrigerate until required.

Nutrition:

Calories:90;

Carbohydrates: 6g;

Protein: 9.4g;

Fat: 1.5g;

Sugar: 0.2g;

Sodium: 671mg;

Fiber: 3g

128.   Porridge

Preparation Time: 5 minutes

Cooking Time: 10 minutes

Servings: 4

Ingredients:

6 Medjool dates, pitted, sliced

5 cardamom pods

1 teaspoon ginger powder

1/8 teaspoon salt

1/4 teaspoon ground nutmeg

2 tablespoons brown sugar

1 teaspoon cinnamon powder

1/4 teaspoon Allspice powder

1 teaspoon vanilla extract, unsweetened

1 cup almond milk, unsweetened

1 cup coconut milk, unsweetened

1 1/2 cups water

Fresh mixed berries for topping

Chopped nuts for topping

Hemp seeds for topping

Coconut flakes for topping

Directions:

Switch on the instant pot, place all the ingredients into the inner pot, except for the garnishing ones, stir until well mixed, and shut the pot with the lid in the sealed position.

Press the manual button, press the +/- button to set the cooking time to 10 minutes, press the pressure level to select the high-pressure setting, and let cook; the instant pot will take 10 minutes to preheat and then the timer will start.

When it's done and the timer beeps, release the pressure through natural pressure release for 5 minutes, then do quick pressure release and carefully move the vent to "venting."

Open the instant pot, stir the pudding, pour in more milk if required, and top with mixed berries, nuts, hemp seeds, and coconut flakes.

Nutrition:

Calories:430;

Carbohydrates:8 g;

Protein: 29g;

Fat: 13.2g;

Sugar: 0.7g;

Sodium: 303mg;

Fiber: 2g

129.   Choco Cake

Preparation Time: 10 minutes

Cooking Time: 35 minutes

Servings: 4

Ingredients:

¾ cup all-purpose flour

½ teaspoon baking soda

¼ teaspoon salt

¼ cup cocoa powder, unsweetened

½ teaspoon baking powder

½ cup of coconut sugar

½ teaspoon vanilla extract, unsweetened

¼ cup olive oil

1 teaspoon apple cider vinegar

½ cup almond milk

Directions:

Take a bowl, add all the dry ingredients in it and stir until mixed, set aside until required.

Take another bowl, pour in milk, stir in vinegar, and let the mixture stand for 1 minute.

Then whip in sugar for 1 minute until sugar has melted, whisk in oil along with remaining ingredients, and gradually beat in the dry ingredients mixture until incorporated and a smooth batter comes together.

Take a 6 by 3-inch metal pan, create a foil sling, place pan in the center, pour in prepared batter, smooth the top, and cover the pan with foil.

Switch on the instant pot, pour water in the inner pot, insert trivet stand, place pan on it with the help of sling, and shut the pot with the lid in the sealed position.

Press the manual button, press the +/- button to set the cooking time to 35 minutes, press the pressure level to select the high-pressure setting, and let cook; the instant pot will take 10 minutes to preheat and then the timer will start.

When it's done and the timer beeps, release the pressure through natural pressure release; this will take 10 minutes, and then carefully move the vent to "venting."

Open the instant pot, take out the cake pan, uncover it, let it cool for 5 minutes, and then take it out.

Transfer cake to cool completely, then cut it into slices and serve.

Nutrition:

Calories:326;

Carbohydrates: 12g;

Protein: 26g;

Fat: 15g;

Sugar: 3g;

Sodium: 890mg;

Fiber: 0g

130. Apple Crumble

Preparation Time: 10 minutes

Cooking Time: 35 minutes

Servings: 4

Ingredients:

5 medium honey crisp apples, peeled, cut into chunks

3/4 cup quick oats

1/4 cup coconut sugar

1/4 cup spelt flour

1/2 teaspoon salt

1 tablespoon maple syrup

2 teaspoons cinnamon

1/4 cup melted coconut oil

1/2 cup water

Directions:

Take a bowl, add oats and flour into it, stir in salt and sugar until mixed, drizzle oil over the mixture, and then stir until well coated, set aside until required.

Switch on the instant pot, place apples in the inner pot, sprinkle with cinnamon, and drizzle with maple syrup.

Pour in water, cover apples with prepared oats mixture, and shut the pot with the lid in the sealed position.

Press the manual button, press the +/- button to set the cooking time 8 minutes, press the pressure level to select the high-pressure setting, and let cook; the instant pot will take 10 minutes to preheat and then the timer will start.

When it's done and the timer beeps, release the pressure through natural pressure release; this will take 10 minutes, and then carefully move the vent to "venting."

Open the instant pot, stir the crisp and transfer them to a dish. Serve apple crisp with ice cream.

Nutrition:Calories:370;Carbohydrates: 12g; Protein: 34g; Fat: 6g; Sugar: 4g; Sodium: 342mg; Fiber: 0g

131. Apple Cake

Preparation Time: 15 minutes

Cooking Time: 50 minutes

Servings: 8

Ingredients:

1 medium banana, peeled, mashed

1 medium apple, peeled, cubed

1 1/2 cup water

Ice cream for serving

2 tablespoons almond flour

1/4 teaspoon cinnamon

1 tablespoon sugar

1/2 cup almond flour

1 cup brown rice flour

2 tablespoons ground flaxseeds

1/4 teaspoon salt

1 tablespoon baking powder

1/4 teaspoon nutmeg

1/2 cup rolled oats

1/2 teaspoon cinnamon

3/4 cup sugar

2 teaspoons vanilla extract, unsweetened

1 cup almond milk, unsweetened

Directions:

Prepare the crumb topping and for this, take a bowl, place all ingredients in it and stir until mixed, then set aside until required.

Prepare the cake and for this, take another bowl, add banana, flaxseeds, and vanilla in it, pour in milk, and stir until combined. Take a large bowl, add both flour and oats in it, stir in flaxseed, sugar, salt, cinnamon, baking powder, and nutmeg in it until combined and then whisk in milk until incorporated.

Add apples and mashed bananas, fold until just mixed, then take a 6-inches cake pan, line with parchment paper, grease it with oil, pour in batter, top with the prepared crumb topping and then cover the pan with foil.

Switch on the instant pot, pour in water, insert the trivet stand, place pan on it, and shut the pot with the lid in the sealed position.

Press the manual button, press the +/- button to set the cooking time to 50 minutes, press the pressure level to select the high-pressure setting, and let cook; the instant pot will take 10 minutes to preheat and then the timer will start.

When it's done and the timer beeps, release the pressure through natural pressure release; this will take 10 minutes, and then carefully move the vent to "venting."

Open the instant pot, take out the pan, uncover it, let it cool for 10 minutes, then transfer pan onto the wire rack and let it cool completely.

Slice the cake and serve with ice cream.

Nutrition:

Calories:100;

Carbohydrates: 13g;

Protein: 24g;

Fat: 11g;

Sugar: 6g;

Sodium: 602mg;

Fiber: 3g

132. Chickpea Slices

Preparation Time: 10 minutes

Cooking Time: 35 minutes

Servings: 4

Ingredients:

4 flour tortillas

½ cup chickpeas, soaked

2 cups of water

1 teaspoon salt

1 tablespoon vegan mayonnaise

1 bell pepper, chopped

Directions:

Place tortillas and chickpeas in the instant pot.

Close and seal the lid.

Cook the chickpeas on Manual mode for 35 minutes. Use quick pressure release.

Drain the water and transfer the chickpeas in the blender.

Add salt, vegan mayonnaise, and bell pepper.

Blend the mixture.

Spread the flour tortillas with the blended chickpeas and roll them.

Slice the tortillas into small pieces and secure with toothpicks.

Nutrition:

Calories:162;

Carbohydrates: 14g;

Protein: 28g;

Fat: 3.1g;

Sugar: 3g;

Sodium: 654mg;

Fiber: 0g

133. Crunchy Oyster Mushrooms

Preparation Time: 15 minutes

Cooking Time: 15 minutes

Servings: 4

Ingredients:

7 oz oyster mushrooms

1 tablespoon olive oil

1 teaspoon chili flakes

¼ cup bread crumbs

1 teaspoon apple cider vinegar

1 cup water, for cooking

Directions:

Place oyster mushrooms in instant pot pan.

Pour water in the instant pot and insert trivet.

Place pan with oyster mushrooms on the trivet and close the lid.

Seal the lid and cook mushrooms for 10 minutes.

After this, use quick pressure release.

Open the lid and drain water.

Chop the oyster mushrooms roughly and sprinkle with olive oil, chili flakes, and apple cider vinegar.

Mix up the mushrooms and let them for 10 minutes to marinate.

Then preheat instant pot on Saute mode.

Add oyster mushrooms and cook them for 4 minutes.

Stir the vegetables and sprinkle with bread crumbs. Mix up the mushrooms well.

Transfer them in the serving bowl.

Nutrition:

Calories:312;

Carbohydrates: 5.2g;

Protein: 20.4g;

Fat: 5.2g;

Sugar: 3g;

Sodium: 1121mg;

Fiber: 3g

134.   Jackfruit Coated Bites

Preparation Time: 15 minutes

Cooking Time: 5 minutes

Servings: 4

Ingredients:

1 cup jackfruit, canned, drained

½ cup wheat flour

2 tablespoons soy sauce

2 tablespoons maple syrup

4 tablespoons agave syrup

1 teaspoon ground cumin

½ teaspoon salt

1 teaspoon paprika

½ teaspoon ground black pepper

1 teaspoon dried cilantro

1 teaspoon turmeric

½ cup olive oil

Directions:

In the mixing bowl, mix up together soy sauce, maple syrup, agave syrup, ground cumin, salt, and paprika. Whisk the mixture.

Place canned jackfruit in the soy mixture and mix up well. Leave it for 10 minutes to marinate. Meanwhile, pour olive oil in the instant pot and preheat it on Saute mode.

In the separated bowl, combine together wheat flour, ground black pepper, cilantro, and turmeric.

Coat the jackfruit into the wheat mixture.

Place the coated pieces of jackfruit in the hot olive oil and cook them for 1 minute from each side or until light brown.

Dry the snack with the paper towel and transfer on the serving bowl

Nutrition:

Calories:412;

Carbohydrates: 3g;

Protein: 35g;

Fat: 7g; Sugar: 1g;

Sodium: 755mg;

Fiber: 1g

135. Sofritas Tofu

Preparation Time: 5 minutes

Cooking Time: 5 minutes

Servings: 4

Ingredients:

8 oz firm tofu, chopped

½ teaspoon cayenne pepper

1 teaspoon ground black pepper

1 teaspoon smoked paprika

1 teaspoon chili flakes

½ teaspoon salt

½ teaspoon brown sugar

1 tablespoon avocado oil

5 tablespoons vegan Adobo sauce

Directions:

Pour avocado oil in the instant pot. Add chopped tofu.

Cook it on Saute mode for 1 minute.

Sprinkle tofu with cayenne pepper, ground black pepper, smoked paprika, chili flakes, and salt. Mix up well and add sugar.

Stir it carefully and cook for 2 minutes.

Then add vegan Adobo sauce and mix up the meal well.

Cook it for 2 minutes more.

Transfer cooked sofritas tofu in the serving bowl.

Nutrition:

Calories:165;

Carbohydrates: 13.4g;

Protein: 4.5g;

Fat: 6g;

Sugar: 0g;

Sodium: 543mg;

Fiber: 1.7g

136. Garlic Pumpkin Seeds

Preparation Time: 5 minutes

Cooking Time: 10 minutes

Servings: 6

Ingredients:

1 ½ cup pumpkin seeds

3 teaspoons garlic powder

½ teaspoon chipotle chili pepper

1 teaspoon salt

1 tablespoon olive oil

Directions:

Place pumpkin seeds in the instant pot.

Set Saute mode and cook them for 5 minutes. Stir pumpkin seeds every 1 minute.

After this, sprinkle the seeds with olive oil, chipotle chili pepper, salt, and garlic powder.

Mix up well and cook for 4 minutes more.

Then switch off the instant pot and let seeds rest for 1 minute.

Nutrition:

Calories:212;

Carbohydrates: 4.5g;

Protein: 8.7g;

Fat: 6g;

Sugar: 2.2g;

Sodium: 456mg;

Fiber: 1g

137.   Polenta Fries

Preparation Time: 15 minutes

Cooking Time: 10 minutes

Servings: 10

Ingredients:

1 cup polenta

3 cups almond milk

1 teaspoon salt

1 teaspoon ground black pepper

1 teaspoon dried cilantro

½ teaspoon ground cumin

1 tablespoon almond butter

1 tablespoon olive oil

Directions:

Place polenta in the instant pot.

Add almond milk and salt.

Then add ground black pepper, dried cilantro, and ground cumin. Mix it up.

Close and seal the lid.

Cook polenta for 6 minutes on High-pressure mode. Allow natural pressure release for 10 minutes.

Open the lid and add almond butter. Mix up it well.

Transfer the polenta into the square pan and flatten well.

Let it chill until solid.

Then cut solid polenta onto 10 sticks.

Brush every stick with the olive oil.

Clean and preheat instant pot on Saute mode until hot.

Then cook polenta sticks for 1 minute from each side or until light brown.

Chill the snack before serving.

Nutrition:

Calories:244;

Carbohydrates: 6.5g;

Protein: 29.4g;

Fat: 14.3g;

Sugar: 0.4g;

Sodium: 564mg;

Fiber: 3.2g

138. Green Croquettes

Preparation Time: 15 minutes

Cooking Time: 5 minutes

Servings: 4

Ingredients:

2 sweet potatoes, peeled, boiled

1 cup fresh spinach

1 tablespoons peanuts

3 tablespoons flax meal

1 teaspoon salt

1 teaspoon ground black pepper

1 tablespoon olive oil

½ teaspoon dried oregano

¾ cup wheat flour

Directions:

Mash the sweet potatoes and place them in the mixing bowl.

Add flax meal salt, dried oregano, and ground black pepper.

Then blend the spinach with peanuts until smooth.

Add the green mixture in the sweet potato.

Mix up the mass.

Make medium size croquettes and coat them in the wheat flour.

Preheat instant pot on Saute mode well.

Add olive oil.

Roast croquettes for 1 minute from each side or until golden brown.

Dry the cooked croquettes with a paper towel if needed.

Nutrition:

Calories:155;

Carbohydrates: 12g;

Protein: 29.4g;

Fat: 6.8g;

Sugar: 4g;

Sodium: 645mg;

Fiber: 7g

139.   Cigar Borek

Preparation Time: 10 minutes

Cooking Time: 5 minutes

Servings: 6

Ingredients:

6 oz phyllo dough

8 oz vegan Parmesan, grated

1 tablespoon vegan mayonnaise

1 teaspoon minced garlic

1 tablespoon avocado oil

Directions:

In the mixing bowl, mix up together grated Parmesan, vegan mayonnaise, and minced garlic.

Then cut phyllo dough into triangles.

Spread the triangles with cheese mixture and roll in the shape of cigars.

Preheat avocado oil in the instant pot on Saute mode.

Place rolled "cigar" in the instant pot and cook them for 1-2 minutes or until they are golden brown.

Nutrition:

Calories:210;

Carbohydrates: 11g;

Protein: 17g;

Fat: 3g;

Sugar: 2.2g;

Sodium: 654mg;

Fiber: 0g

Smoothie Recipes

140. Crisp Cucumber Mango Green Smoothie

Preparation Time: 5 minutes

Cooking Time: 0 minutes

Servings: 1

Ingredients

Orange – 1 (peeled)

Mango - ¼ cup

Flax seeds - 1 tablespoon

Chopped cucumber - 1 cup

Spinach - 1 cup

Directions

Add all the smoothie ingredients into your blender and puree until creamy and smooth.

Enjoy!

Nutrition:

Calories:269;

Carbohydrates: 8.6g;

Protein: 7.1g;

Fat: 25.9g;

Sugar: 0.8g;

Sodium: 161mg;

Fiber: 5.7g

141. Green Tropical Surprise

Preparation Time: 5 minutes

Cooking Time: 0 minutes

Servings: 1

Ingredients Carrot – 1

Orange – 1 (peeled)

Pineapple - ¼ cup

Flax seeds - 1 tablespoon

Spinach - 1 cup

Water - 1 cup

Directions Add all the smoothie ingredients into your blender and puree until creamy and smooth. Enjoy!

Nutrition: Calories:134;

Carbohydrates: 10g;

Protein: 4.6g; Fat: 8.8g;

Sugar: 2.6g; Sodium: 110mg;

Fiber: 3.8g

142. Banana Spinach Smoothie

Preparation Time: 5 minutes

Cooking Time: 0 minutes

Servings: 1

Ingredients

Wheat Germ or Ground Flax Seed - 1 teaspoon

Soy or skim milk - 1 cup

Whole Banana – 1 (Sliced)

Fresh Baby Spinach Leaves - 1 cup (Packed)

Crushed Ice - ½ cups

Directions

Add all the ingredients in a blender or Magic bullet. Blend until smooth, about 30 seconds. Pour into a glass.

Enjoy!

Nutrition:

Calories:383;

Carbohydrates: 4.4g;

Protein: 14.8g;

Fat: 28.4g;

Sugar: 2g;

Sodium: 379mg; Fiber: 1.2g

143. Tropical Green Paleo Smoothie

Preparation Time: 15 minutes

Cooking Time: 0 minutes

Servings: 5

Ingredients

Spinach - 3 cups (Kale, or a blend of small leafy greens, packed)

Whole Banana – 1 (Peeled)

Whole Orange – 1 (Peeled)

Pineapple - 1-½ cup (Cubed)

Coconut Milk - 1 cup

Whole Avocado - ½ (pitted and skin removed)

Crushed Ice - 2 cups

Wild Orange Essential Oil - 3 drops (optional)

Dried Coconut Chips - 10 pieces (optional)

Dried Coconut Chips, For Topping (optional)

Pure Maple Syrup - 1 Tablespoon (optional, depends on the sweetness of fruit)

Chia Seeds, For Topping - 1 teaspoon (optional)

Directions

Add all the ingredients minus the chia seeds and coconut chips in a high-speed blender. Blend for about 2 minutes, until its creamy and smooth.

Transfer mixture to serving glasses and top with the chia seeds and coconut seeds. It can be refrigerated for up to 3 days. Stir quickly to recombine if placed in the fridge.

Nutrition:

Calories:33;

Carbohydrates: 8.5g;

Protein: 2.2g;

Fat: 0.4g;

Sugar: 4.3g;

Sodium: 225mg;

Fiber: 1.9g

144. Vegan Banana Avocado Green Smoothie Bowl with Blueberries

Preparation Time: 5 minutes

Cooking Time: 0 minutes

Servings: 1

Ingredients

For the Smoothie

Fresh Baby Spinach - 60 grams

Whole Avocado - ½

Whole Peach – 1

Whole Banana - ½

Rolled Oats - 2 Tablespoons

Peanut Butter - 1 Tablespoon

Coconut Water - 3 Tablespoons

For the Topping

whole Blueberries – 12

Cacao Nibs - 1 teaspoon

Directions

Add all the smoothie ingredients in your blender. Blend until creamy and smooth, about 30 seconds.

Pour into a bowl and add toppings.

Enjoy!

Nutrition:

Calories:414;

Carbohydrates: 10.8g;

Protein: 12.5g;

Fat: 35.7g;

Sugar: 0.6g;

Sodium: 188mg;

Fiber: 4.8g

145. Kale Strawberry Green Smoothie Bowl

Preparation Time: 8 minutes

Cooking Time: 0 minutes

Servings: 1

Ingredients

For the Smoothie

Whole Strawberries – 2

Zucchini – 2 ounces

Kale - 1 cup

Sliced Cucumber – 1.4 ounces

Whole Banana - ½

Dairy-Free Milk - 4 tablespoons

For the Topping

Whole Strawberry – 1

Hemp Hearts - ½ Tablespoon

Shredded Coconut - 1 Tablespoon

Whole Oats - 2 Tablespoons

Directions

Add all the smoothie ingredients to a high-speed blender. Blend for about 2 minutes, until it is creamy and smooth.

Transfer the mixture to serving bowls and add the toppings.

Nutrition:

Calories:326;

Carbohydrates: 8.2g;

Protein: 7.8g;

Fat: 29.4g;

Sugar: 0.3g;

Sodium: 126mg;

Fiber: 4.1g

146. Spirulina Green Smoothie Bowl

Preparation Time: 5 minutes

Cooking Time: 0 minutes

Servings: 1

Ingredients

For the Smoothie

Frozen Uncooked Cauliflower - 2-½ ounces

Banana - ½

Peach – 1

Spirulina Powder - 1 teaspoon

Rolled Oats - 3 Tablespoons

Nondairy Milk - 4 tablespoons

For the Topping

Fresh Raspberries - 8

Fresh Fig – 1

Coconut Flakes - ¼ ounces

Cacao Nibs - ⅛ ounces

Directions

Add all the smoothie ingredients to a high-speed blender. Blend for about 2 minutes, until it is creamy and smooth.

Transfer the mixture to serving bowls and add the toppings.

Nutrition:

Calories:249;

Carbohydrates: 7.1g;

Protein: 5.6g;

Fat: 22.8g;

Sugar: 0.7g;

Sodium: 183mg;

Fiber: 4g

147. Avocado Spinach Green Smoothie Bowl

Preparation Time: 5 minutes

Cooking Time: 0 minutes

Servings: 1

Ingredients

For the Smoothie

Fresh Baby Spinach - 2 cups

Kiwi – 1

Avocado - ½

Strawberries – 2

Dairy-Free Milk – 3 tablespoons

Peanut Butter - 1 Tablespoon

Rolled Oats - 5 Tablespoons

Directions

Add all the smoothie ingredients to a high-speed blender. Blend for about 2 minutes, until it is creamy and smooth.

Transfer the mixture to serving bowls and add your preferred toppings.

Nutrition:

Calories:414;

Carbohydrates: 10.8g;

Protein: 12.5g;

Fat: 35.7g;

Sugar: 0.6g;

Sodium: 188mg;

Fiber: 4.8g

148. Matcha Smoothie

Preparation Time: 5 minutes

Cooking Time: 0 minutes

Servings: 1

Ingredients

Frozen Pineapple - 1 cup

Greens, like kale or spinach - ⅓ cup

Avocado - ½ cup

Coconut or almond - ½ cup

Banana – ½

Matcha Powder - 2 teaspoons

Directions Add all the smoothie ingredients to a high-speed blender. Blend for about 2 minutes, until it is creamy and smooth. Add more milk if it is too thick; add another half banana or more ice if it is too thin. Enjoy!

Nutrition: Calories:134;

Carbohydrates: 10g;

Protein: 4.6g; Fat: 8.8g;

Sugar: 2.6g; Sodium: 110mg;

Fiber: 3.8g

149. Spinach Papaya Green Smoothie Bowl

Preparation Time: 5 minutes

Cooking Time: 0 minutes

Servings: 1

Ingredients

For the Smoothie

Raw Spinach - 1 cup

Papaya - 1 cup

Peach – 1

Rolled Oats - 3 Tablespoons

Ground Flax Seeds – 1 Tablespoon

Non-dairy Milk - 3 Tablespoons

For the Topping

Coconut Flakes - ¼ ounces

Blackberries –4

Cacao Nibs - ¼ ounces

Directions

Add all the smoothie ingredients to a high-speed blender. Blend for about 1 minute, until it is creamy and smooth.

Transfer the mixture to your serving bowl, then add the toppings.

Nutrition:

Calories:249;

Carbohydrates: 7.1g;

Protein: 5.6g;

Fat: 22.8g;

Sugar: 0.7g;

Sodium: 183mg;

Fiber: 4g

150. Green Smoothie

Preparation Time: 5 minutes

Cooking Time: 0 minutes

Servings: 2

Ingredients

For the Smoothie

Baby Kale - 3 cups

Cashews - 3 Tablespoons

Banana - ½

Ginger - 1 teaspoon

Milk - ½ cup

Vanilla Extract - ½ teaspoon

Maple Syrup - ½ Tablespoon

Ice Cubes - ¾ cup

Directions

First, add the cashews, baby kale, ginger, and banana to your blender. Followed by the vanilla extract, maple syrup, milk, and ice cubes.

Blend for about 45 seconds, until you get a smooth blend.

Nutrition:

Calories:383;

Carbohydrates: 4.4g;

Protein: 14.8g;

Fat: 28.4g;

Sugar: 2g;

Sodium: 379mg;

Fiber: 1.2g

151. Pear Banana Spinach Smoothie Bowl

Preparation Time: 10 minutes

Cooking Time: 0 minutes

Servings: 1

Ingredients

For the Smoothie

Banana - ½

Medium-size Pear - 1

Ground Oats - 3 Tablespoons

Fresh Baby Spinach - 1 cup

Fresh Water – 3 ½ tablespoons

For the Topping

Banana - ½ (Sliced)

Coconut Flakes - 1 teaspoon

Peanut Butter - 1 teaspoon

Hemp Hearts - ⅓ teaspoons

Directions

Add all the smoothie ingredients to a high-speed blender. Blend for about 1 minute, until it is creamy and smooth.

Transfer the mixture to your serving bowl, then add the toppings.

Nutrition:

Calories:198;

Carbohydrates: 10.1g;

Protein: 6.5g;

Fat: 15g;

Sugar: 1.6g; Sodium: 73mg;

Fiber: 5.4g

152. Mixed Greens Smoothie Bowl

Preparation Time: 5 minutes

Cooking Time: 0 minutes

Servings: 1

Ingredients

Banana - ½ (peeled)

Fresh Mixed Greens - 1 cup

Medium Size Strawberries - 3

Fresh Baby Spinach - ½ cup

Flaxseed Meal - 1 Tablespoon

Hemp Protein - 1 teaspoon

Maca Powder - 1 teaspoon

Nondairy Milk - 7 Tablespoons

Rolled Oats - 3 Tablespoons

Directions   Add   all   the smoothie ingredients to a high-speed blender. Blend for about 1 minute, until it is creamy and smooth.

Transfer the mixture to serving bowl and add your preferred toppings. Enjoy!

Nutrition: Calories: 453

Fat: 33.4 g Protein: 19.1 g

Net Carbs: 5.5 g Fiber: 3.75 g

153. Vegan Green Smoothie Bowl

Preparation Time: 10 minutes

Cooking Time: 0 minutes

Servings: 1

Ingredients

For the Smoothie

Fresh Pineapple - 2 ounces

Broccoli Florets - 2-⅛ ounces

Small Cucumber - ½ (chopped)

Fresh Parsley - 1 cup

Peanut Butter - 1 Tablespoon

Water - 2 tablespoons

Spinach - 1 leaf

For the Topping

Goji Berries - 1 Tablespoon

Hazelnuts and sliced walnuts - ½ Tablespoon

Chia Seeds - 1 Tablespoon

Hemp Hearts - ½ teaspoon

Directions

Add   all   the   smoothie ingredients   to   a   high-speed blender. Blend until it is creamy and smooth.

Transfer mixture to a serving bowl, add your toppings, and stir the content together. Allow to sit for approx. 30 minutes so that the chia seeds can expand.

Nutrition:

Calories:365;

Carbohydrates: 5.6g;

Protein: 12g; Fat: 33.6g;

Sugar: 3g;

Sodium: 373mg;

Fiber: 1.8g

154. Minty Alkaline Kiwi Green Smoothie

Preparation Time: 10 minutes

Cooking Time: 0 minutes

Servings: 2

Ingredients

Kiwi – 1 (sliced in half & flesh scooped out)

English Cucumber - ½ (Diced with skin On)

Pink or green lady apple – 1 (Peeled And Sliced)

Spinach - 1 cup (Tightly Packed)

Pure Honey – 2 teaspoons

Fresh Mint - 10 leaves

Banana – 1

Lemon Zest - 1 teaspoon

Raw Coconut Oil - 1 Tablespoon (optional)

Medium Lemon - ½ (Juiced)

Water - ¼ cup

Directions

Add all the ingredients in your blender to blitz for about 30 to 60 seconds or until creamy and smooth.

Add an extra banana or more honey if you want more sweetness in the smoothie. Drink.

Stew Recipes

155. Beef And Cabbage Stew

Preparation Time: 15 minutes

Cooking Time: 10 minutes

Servings: 6

Ingredients

1 1/2 lbs. beef stew meat, cut into 1-inch pieces

1 cube beef bouillon

2 cups beef broth

1 large onion, chopped

1/4 tsp. ground black pepper

1 bay leaf

2 potatoes, peeled and cubed

4 cups shredded cabbage

2 celery ribs, sliced

1 carrot, sliced

1 (8 oz.) can tomato sauce

salt to taste

Direction

In the Dutch oven or a large saucepan, cook and mix stew meat over medium heat for 10 - 15 minutes, until all sides are browned evenly. Drain off excess grease.

In a bowl, stir beef broth and beef bouillon together until dissolved; spread over stew meat. Add bay leaf, black pepper, and onion; simmer while covered for 2 hours or more, until stew meat is softened. Add carrot, celery, cabbage, and potatoes; simmer while covered for 30 - 45 minutes more, until potatoes get softened.

Whisk salt and tomato sauce into the stew; simmer while uncovered for 15 to 20 minutes, up to tomato sauce is well incorporated and flavors are blended properly.

Nutrition:

Calories:365;

Carbohydrates: 5.6g;

Protein: 12g; Fat: 33.6g;

Sugar: 3g;

Sodium: 373mg; Fiber: 1.8g

156. German Sauerbraten Stew

Preparation Time: 20 minutes

Cooking Time:2hours 20 minutes

Servings: 14

Ingredients

2 lbs. boneless pork, trimmed and cut into 1-1/2-inch cubes

2 tbsps. vegetable oil

1-1/2 quarts water

2 cups ketchup

1 large onion, chopped

2 medium potatoes, peeled and cubed

3 medium carrots, cut into 1/2-in slices

1 cup fresh or frozen cut green beans (1-inch pieces)

1 cup shredded cabbage

2 celery ribs, cut into 1/2-inch slices

1/4 to 1/2 tsp. ground allspice

1/4 tsp. pepper

1 cup crushed gingersnaps (about 16 cookies)

Direction

Cook pork in oil in a soup kettle or Dutch oven until browned. Put the next 10 ingredients into the pan. Simmer, covered for 1 hour and 30 minutes. Mix in gingersnap crumbs; simmer without covering until pork is tender and stew thickens, or for 30 minutes

Nutrition:

Calories:215;

Carbohydrates: 24g;

Protein: 12g;

Fat: 23.6g;

Sugar: 1g;

Sodium: 208mg;

Fiber: 1.0g

157.   Lemon And Tomato Fish Stew

Preparation Time: 30 minutes

Cooking Time: 1hour 35 minutes

Servings: 4

Ingredients

1 cup brown rice

2 tbsps. olive oil

1/2 onion, chopped

1 stalk celery, finely chopped

4 cloves garlic, chopped

1 Hatch chile pepper, seeded and chopped

1 Roma tomato, chopped

1 1/2 tbsps. tomato paste

1 cup chicken broth

1/2 cup white wine

2 bay leaves

1 tbsp. butter

2 salmon fillets

salt and ground black pepper to taste

1/4 cup sour cream

1 tbsp. lemon juice, or to taste

1 bunch green onions, chopped

Direction

Boil water and brown rice in a saucepan. Bring the heat to medium-low, cover the pan and let to simmer for about 45 to 50 minutes until the liquid is absorbed and the rice becomes tender.

On high heat, heat oil in a deep skillet and add garlic, onion, and celery. Cook while stirring for about 5 minutes until the edges of onion turn brown. Stir in tomato paste, tomato, and chile pepper. Cook while stirring continuously for 1 minute until softened.

Mix bay leaves, white wine, and chicken broth into the skillet and simmer for 5 minutes until the stew is evenly warmed.

On medium heat, melt butter in a pot and add salmon. Add pepper and salt to taste. Cook for about 3 to 5 minutes on each side, turning once, until the salmon easily flakes with a fork. Divide into small pieces.

Mix lemon juice and sour cream into the stew and spread the stew atop salmon. Take out bay leaves and place in green onions.

Separate the brown rice evenly into four bowls. Spoon the stew atop rice.

Nutrition:

Calories:445;

Carbohydrates: 6g;

Protein: 12g;

Fat: 17.6g;

Sugar: 3g;

Sodium: 402mg;

Fiber: 1.8g

158. Ground Beef Stew

Preparation Time: 15 minutes

Cooking Time: 6hours 10 minutes

Servings: 6

Ingredients

2 large potatoes, sliced

2 medium carrots, sliced

1 can (15 oz.) peas, drained

3 medium onions, sliced

2 celery ribs, sliced

1-1/2 lbs. ground beef, cooked and drained

1 can (10-3/4 oz.) condensed tomato soup, undiluted

1-1/3 cups water

Direction

In a 5-quart slow cooker, put the first six ingredients listed in order in layers. In a tiny bowl, mix water and soup together. Spread over beef.

Cook on low while covered for 6-8 hours, until vegetables are softened.

Nutrition:

Calories:385;

Carbohydrates: 46g;

Protein: 27g;

Fat: 11g;

Sugar: 1g;

Sodium: 580mg;

Fiber: 7g

159.   Beef Stew With Cheddar Dumplings

Preparation Time: 25 minutes

Cooking Time: 1hour 55 minutes

Servings: 8

Ingredients

1/2 cup all-purpose flour

1/2 tsp. salt

1/2 tsp. pepper

2 to 3 lbs. beef stew meat, cut into 1-inch pieces

2 tbsps. canola oil

5 cups water

5 tsps. beef bouillon granules

1 tbsp. browning sauce, optional

1/2 tsp. onion salt

1/2 tsp. garlic salt

4 medium carrots, sliced

1 medium onion, cut into wedges

1 can (14-1/2 oz.) cut green beans, drained

DUMPLINGS:

2 cups biscuit/baking mix

1 cup shredded cheddar cheese

2/3 cup whole milk

Direction

Combine pepper, salt, and flour in a large resealable plastic bag. Add a few pieces of beef at a time to the bag and shake to coat until finished. Cook beef in oil in batches in a Dutch oven until browned.

Mix in bouillon, water, garlic salt, onion salt, and browning sauce if desired. Bring to a boil. Lower heat; simmer, covered, for 1 hour.

Add onion and carrots. Simmer, covered, until vegetables are softened, about 10 to 15 minutes more. Mix in green beans.

To make dumplings, mix together cheese and biscuit mix. Add enough milk to the mixture, stirring until a soft dough is formed. Drop tablespoonfuls of the dough onto simmering stew. Simmer, covered, until a toothpick comes out clean from the center of the dumplings, about 10 to 12 minutes (do not peek while dumplings are being cooked). Serve right away.

Nutrition:

Calories:441;

Carbohydrates: 33g;

Protein: 30g;

Fat: 21g;

Sugar: 3g;

Sodium: 1627mg;

Fiber: 3g

160.   Irish Stew With Pearl Barley

Preparation Time: 15 minutes

Cooking Time: 20 minutes

Servings: 4

Ingredients

4 (12-oz., 1 1/4-inch–thick) bone-in lamb leg chops (3 lb. total)

Salt and freshly ground black pepper

9 oz. carrots (about 5 small carrots scrubbed and halved at an angle, or 3 large carrots, peeled and cut at an angle into 1 1/2-inch pieces)

9 oz. celery (about 4 stalks), trimmed and cut at an angle into 1 1/2-inch pieces

3 onions, peeled and each cut into 6 wedges

8 large cloves of garlic, peeled and left whole

1/4 cup pearl barley

2 1/2 cups lamb or chicken stock

8–12 potatoes

2 tbsps. chopped parsley leaves

Direction

Turn oven to 325°F to preheat. Place a large saucepan or a flameproof casserole on a medium-high heat. Trim the excess fat from the chops and put the scraps of fat into the pan to render.

In the meantime, cut chops in half lengthwise in order not to go through the bone. Once some fat has melted, take out and discard the unmelted or unrendered ones. Enjoy eat or feed your dog. Raise the heat to high and put the chops into the pan. Cook both sides, seasoning with pepper and salt, until both sides are browned, take out and place onto a plate.

Add garlic, onions, celery, and carrots to the pan, sprinkle with pepper and salt to season and stir well on the heat until edges starts to turn golden slightly, for a few minutes. Add meat (and all the juices) back to the pan along with stock and barley; mix well to combine. Bring the mixture to a boil and cook, covered for 1 hour in the oven.

In the meantime, peel off potato skin and cut in half if big. Once 1 hour is over, remove the pan from the oven and add potatoes on top. Cover and return to the oven; bake until cooked, for 35 to 45 minutes. Sprinkle with parsley and serve right from the pan.

Nutrition:

Calories:908;

Carbohydrates: 128g;

Protein: 38g;

Fat: 33.6g;

Sugar: 3g;

Sodium: 2373mg;

Fiber: 12g

161. Hearty Beef & Sweet Potato Stew

Preparation Time: 2hours 40 minutes

Cooking Time: 20 minutes

Servings: 8

Ingredients

3 tbsps. canola oil, divided

1-1/2 lbs. boneless beef chuck steak, cut into 1-inch pieces

2 medium onions, chopped

2 garlic cloves, minced

2 cans (14-1/2 oz. each) reduced-sodium beef broth

1/3 cup dry red wine or additional reduced-sodium beef broth

1 tbsp. minced fresh thyme or 1 tsp. dried thyme

1 tbsp. Worcestershire sauce

1 tsp. salt

3/4 tsp. pepper

3 tbsps. cornstarch

3 tbsps. cold water

1-1/4 lbs. sweet potatoes (about 2 medium), cut into 1-inch cubes

1 lb. baby portobello mushrooms, halved

4 medium carrots, cut into 1/2-inch slices

2 medium parsnips, cut into 1/2-inch slices

1 medium turnip, cut into 3/4-inch cubes

Direction

Turn oven to 325° to preheat. Heat 2 tbsps. oil in an oven-safe Dutch oven over medium-high heat. Cook beef in batches until browned. Take cooked beef out using a slotted spoon.

Sauté onions in remaining oil in the pan until softened, or for 2 to 3 minutes. Add garlic, and cook for 1 minute longer. Put in wine and broth, stir to remove browned bits from the pan. Mix in pepper, salt, Worcestershire sauce, and thyme.

Pour beef back to the pan; bring to a boil. Cover and bake for 1 hour and 15 minutes.

Combine cold water and cornstarch together in a small bowl until smooth; slowly mix into stew. Add turnip, parsnips, carrots, mushrooms, and sweet potatoes to the pan. Cover and bake until beef and vegetables are softened, or for 45 minutes to 1 hour longer. Drain cooking juice, if necessary; ladle off fat. Pour cooking juice back in the Dutch oven.

Nutrition:

Calories:354;

Carbohydrates: 4.4g;

Protein: 14.8g;

Fat: 28.4g;

Sugar: 2g;

Sodium: 579mg;

Fiber: 1.2g

162. Cabbage Sausage Stew

Preparation Time: 15 minutes

Cooking Time: 45 minutes

Servings: 8

Ingredients

1 lb. Johnsonville® Fully Cooked Polish Kielbasa Sausage Rope, cut into 3/4-inch pieces

6 medium red potatoes, cut into 3/4-inch chunks

1 small head cabbage, cubed

1 medium onion, cut into 8 wedges

1 tsp. dried oregano

1 tsp. brown sugar, optional

1 tsp. salt, optional

1/8 tsp. pepper

1 can (14-1/2 oz.) stewed tomatoes, undrained

Direction

Cook sausage in a skillet until browned lightly.

Put in onion, cabbage and potatoes. Sprinkle over with

pepper, brown sugar, salt if wanted, and oregano. Put tomatoes on top all; bring to a boil.

Lower heat, then cover and simmer until cabbage and potatoes are softened, about 30 to 35 minutes. Serve in bowls.

Nutrition:

Calories:152;

Carbohydrates: 4.4g;

Protein: 12g;

Fat: 5g;

Sugar: 4g;

Sodium: 234mg;

Fiber: 2.3g

163. Hearty Stew

Preparation Time: 25 minutes

Cooking Time: 15 minutes

Servings: 8

Ingredients

2 lbs. boneless venison or beef chuck roast, cut in 1-inch cubes

2 tbsps. canola oil

4-1/4 cups water, divided

1/2 cup tomato juice

2 medium onions, cut in wedges

2 celery ribs, sliced

1 tsp. Worcestershire sauce

2 bay leaves

2 to 3 tsps. salt

1/2 tsp. pepper

6 medium carrots, quartered

1 large rutabaga, peeled and cubed

6 medium potatoes, peeled and quartered

1 cup frozen peas

1 tbsp. cornstarch

Direction

Brown meat in a Dutch oven with oil on moderate heat.

Put in 4 cups of water and scrape to loosen any browned drippings from pan. Put in pepper, salt, bay leaves, Worcestershire sauce, celery, onions and tomato juice, then bring the mixture to a boil. Lower heat, place a cover and cook while stirring sometimes, about 2 hours.

Get rid of bay leaves, then put in potatoes, rutabaga and carrots. Place a cover and cook about 40 to 60 minutes.

Stir in peas and cook for another 10 minutes. Mix together leftover water and cornstarch until smooth, then stir into the stew. Bring the mixture to a boil, then cook and stir until thickened, about 2 minutes.

Nutrition:

Calories:351;

Carbohydrates: 4.4g;

Protein: 31g;

Fat: 7g;

Sugar: 1g;

Sodium: 234mg;

Fiber: 2.3g

164. Chicken Stew!

Preparation Time: 20 minutes

Cooking Time: 2hours 20 minutes

Servings: 6

Ingredients

4 cups water

1 lb. chicken tenders

3 carrots, cut into chunks

2 stalks celery, cut into chunks

2 potatoes, diced

1 sweet potato, diced

1 (15 oz.) can peas

1 (8 oz.) can tomato sauce

2 bay leaves

1 cup cooked rice

Direction

In a pot, combine bay leaves, tomato sauce, peas, sweet potato, potatoes, celery, carrots, chicken and water; bring to a simmer, lower to medium heat and let simmer for 1 3/4 hours. Mix cooked rice into the soup and cook for about 15 minutes longer until the rice is hot and breaks into grains.

Nutrition:

Calories:273;

Carbohydrates: 4.4g;

Protein: 21.8g;

Fat: 2.4g;

Sugar: 2g;

Sodium: 435mg;

Fiber: 1.2g

165.   Mulligan Stew

Preparation Time: 30 minutes

Cooking Time:3hrs 30 minutes

Servings: 8

Ingredients

1/4 cup all-purpose flour

1 tsp. pepper

1 lb. beef stew meat, cut into 1-inch cubes

1 tbsp. vegetable oil

2 cans (10-1/2 oz. each) beef broth

1 cup water

2 bay leaves

1/2 tsp. garlic salt

1/2 tsp. dried oregano

1/2 tsp. dried basil

1/2 tsp. dill weed

3 medium carrots, cut into 1-inch slices

2 medium potatoes, peeled and cubed

2 celery ribs, cut into 1-inch slices

1 onion, cut into eight wedges

1 cup each frozen corn, green beans, lima beans and peas

1 tbsp. cornstarch

2 tbsps. cold water

1 tbsp. minced fresh parsley

Direction

Combine pepper and flour; roll in beef cubes. Brown beef in the Dutch oven filled with oil. Add dill, basil, oregano, garlic salt, bay leaves, water and broth; allow to boil.

Decrease heat; simmer while covered for about 2 hours until meat is softened.

Add carrots, potatoes, celery and onion; cover and simmer for 40 minutes. Add peas, beans and corn; simmer while covered for 15 minutes more, till vegetables are softened.

Whisk cold water and cornstarch until smooth; move to stew. Allow to boil; boil and stir for around 2 minutes. Throw away bay leaves then put in parsley.

Nutrition:

Calories:203;

Carbohydrates: 25g;

Protein: 11g;

Fat: 18g;

Sugar: 0g;

Sodium: 254mg;

Fiber: 0g

166.   Low-fat Beef Stew

Preparation Time: 20 minutes

Cooking Time: 50 minutes

Servings: 8

Ingredients

1 lb. beef top round steak, trimmed and cubed

1 tsp. canola oil

1 can (14-1/2 oz.) no-salt-added diced tomatoes, undrained

1 cup water

1 tsp. sugar

1/2 tsp. Worcestershire sauce

1/2 tsp. dried thyme

1/4 tsp. pepper

1 bay leaf

4 medium carrots, cut into 3-inch chunks

4 medium potatoes, peeled and halved

1 cup frozen peas

Direction

In a Dutch oven, cook beef in oil until browned.

Add the next 7 ingredients; cook for 10 minutes over medium heat. Add potatoes and carrots; simmer, covered for about half an hour until vegetables are softened.

Remove bay leaf. Mix in peas; cook until thoroughly heated

Nutrition:

Calories:159;

Carbohydrates: 20g;

Protein: 16g;

Fat: 28.4g;

Sugar: 2g;

Sodium: 70mg;

Fiber: 0g

167.   Posse Stew

Preparation Time: 15 minutes

Cooking Time: 1 hour

Servings: 16

Ingredients

1 lb. ground beef

1 (20 oz.) can white or yellow hominy, rinsed and drained

2 (14.5 oz.) cans stewed tomatoes

1 (15.25 oz.) can whole kernel corn

1 (15 oz.) can kidney beans

2 (15 oz.) cans ranch-style beans

1 large yellow onion, chopped

2 green chile peppers, chopped

Direction

In a large frying pan, cook ground beef over medium-high heat while stirring often to crumble, until evenly browned. Drain to remove grease, and shift to a soup pot. Pour in the ranch-style beans, kidney beans, corn, stewed tomatoes, hominy, then add green chilies and onion.

Cook over medium heat while covered for 1 hour.

Nutrition: Calories:547;

Carbohydrates: 4.4g;

Protein: 14.8g; Fat: 1g;

Sugar: 1g; Sodium: 594mg;

Fiber: 1.2g

168.   Onion Meatball Stew

Preparation Time: 20 minutes

Cooking Time: 45 minutes

Servings: 4

Ingredients

1 egg, lightly beaten

1/2 cup soft bread crumbs

1 garlic clove, minced

1/2 tsp. salt

1/2 tsp. dried savory

1 lb. ground beef

1 tbsp. vegetable oil

1 can (10-1/2 oz.) condensed French onion soup, undiluted

2/3 cup water

3 medium carrots, cut into 3/4-inch chunks

2 medium potatoes, peeled and cut into 1-inch chunks

1 medium onion, cut into thin wedges

1 tbsp. minced fresh parsley

Direction

In a big bowl, mix savory, salt, garlic, bread crumbs, and egg together. Crumble beef over the combination and stir properly. Form into 1 - 1/4-inch balls.

In a large frying pan over medium heat, cook meatballs in oil until browned; then drain. Stir in onion, potatoes, carrots, water and soup. Let it boil. Lessen heat, simmer while covered for 25-30 minutes, until vegetables are softened.

Dust with parsley.

Nutrition:

Calories:381;

Carbohydrates: 32g;

Protein: 26g;

Fat: 17g;

Sugar: 2g;

Sodium: 1015mg;

Fiber: 4g

169. Apple Beef Stew

Preparation Time: 10 minutes

Cooking Time: 2hours 05 minutes

Servings: 4

Ingredients

2 lbs. boneless beef chuck roast, cut into 1-inch cubes

2 tbsps. butter

2 medium onions, cut into wedges

2 tbsps. all-purpose flour

1/8 tsp. salt

2 cups water

2 tbsps. apple juice

2 bay leaves

2 whole allspice

2 whole cloves

2 medium carrots, sliced

2 medium apples, peeled and cut into wedges

Directions

In a Dutch oven, brown beef in butter over medium heat. Add onions, cook until turning light brown. Sprinkle salt and flour on top.

Slowly pour in apple juice and water. Boil it, cook while stirring for 2 minutes.

In a double thickness cheesecloth, put cloves, allspice, and bay leaves; lift the corners of the cloth and use a string to tie to make a bag. Put in the pan. Lower the heat, simmer with a cover until the meat is nearly soft, about 1-1/2 hours.

Add apples and carrots, simmer with a cover until the apples, carrots, and meat are soft, about another 15 minutes. Remove the spice bag. Thicken if wanted.

Nutrition:

Calories:526;

Carbohydrates: 22g;

Protein: 46g; Fat: 28g;

Sugar: 2g;

Sodium: 238mg;

Fiber: 4g

Dinner recipes

170.   Lemon-Garlic Chicken Thighs

Preparation Time: 10 minutes

Cooking Time: 25 minutes

Servings: 4

Ingredients

- 4 wedges lemon
- ¼ cup lemon juice
- 4 chicken thighs
- 2 tbsp olive oil
- Pinch ground black pepper
- 1 tsp Dijon mustard
- ¼ tsp salt
- 2 garlic cloves, thinly cut

Directions

Before anything, ensure that your air fryer is preheated 360 degrees F.

Into a medium sized bowl, add lemon juice, pepper, salt, olive oil, garlic, and Dijon mustard. Using a whisk, combine these ingredients and set it aside for a bit. This is your marinade.

You'll need a large resealable plastic bag for this part. Put your chicken thighs and the marinade inside the bag and seal it. Leave it in your refrigerator for about 2 hours.

Next, take the chicken thighs out of the resealable bag, and using a paper towel, dry out the marinade. Place the thighs in an air fryer basket and cook them. You could fry them in batches, if that would make it easier.

When the chicken thighs no longer look pink close to the bone, the frying should last up to 24 minutes in order to achieve this, you can take them out of the air fryer. If you place an instant-read thermometer on the bone, it should read 165 degrees F.

When you serve the chicken thighs, also squeeze the lemon wedges on each of them.

Nutrition:

Calories:258;

Carbohydrates: 3.6g;

Protein: 19.4g;

Fat: 6g;

Sugar: 3g;

Sodium: 242mg;

Fiber: 0g

171.   Black Eyed Peas and Spinach Platter

Preparation Time: 10 minutes

Cooking Time: 8hours

Servings: 4

Ingredients:

1 cup black eyed peas, soaked overnight and drained

2 cups low-sodium vegetable broth

1 can (15 ounces) tomatoes, diced with juice

8 ounces ham, chopped

1 onion, chopped

2 garlic cloves, minced

1 teaspoon dried oregano

1 teaspoon salt

½ teaspoon freshly ground black pepper

½ teaspoon ground mustard

1 bay leaf

Directions:

Add the listed ingredients to your Slow Cooker and stir.

Place lid and cook on LOW for 8 hours.

Discard the bay leaf.

Serve and enjoy!

Nutrition:

Calories:209;

Carbohydrates: 17g;

Protein: 27g;

Fat: 6g;

Sugar: 1.3g;

Sodium: 254mg;

Fiber: 0.5g

172. Humble Mushroom Rice

Preparation Time: 10 minutes

Cooking Time: 3hours

Servings: 3

Ingredients:

½ cup rice

2 green onions chopped

1 garlic clove, minced

¼ pound baby Portobello mushrooms, sliced

1 cup vegetable stock

Directions:

Add rice, onions, garlic, mushrooms, stock to your Slow Cooker.

Stir well and place lid.

Cook on LOW for 3 hours..

Stir and divide amongst serving platters.

Enjoy!

Nutrition: Calories:200;

Carbohydrates: 12g;

Protein: 28g; Fat: 6g;

Sugar: 2.1g;

Sodium: 564mg; Fiber: 0g

173. Sweet and Sour Cabbage and Apples

Preparation Time: 15 minutes

Cooking Time: 8hours 15 minutes

Servings: 4

Ingredients:

¼ cup honey

¼ cup apple cider vinegar

2 tablespoons Orange Chili-Garlic Sauce

1 teaspoon sea salt

3 sweet tart apples, peeled, cored and sliced

2 heads green cabbage, cored and shredded

1 sweet red onion, thinly sliced

Directions:

Take a small bowl and whisk in honey, orange-chili garlic sauce, vinegar.

Stir well.

Add honey mix, apples, onion and cabbage to your Slow Cooker and stir.

Close lid and cook on LOW for 8 hours.

Serve and enjoy!

Nutrition:

Calories:164;

Carbohydrates: 41g;

Protein: 24g;

Fat: 2.5g;

Sugar: 2.4g;

Sodium: 486mg;

Fiber: 3g

174. Orange and Chili Garlic Sauce

Preparation Time: 15 minutes

Cooking Time: 8hours 15 minutes

Servings: 5

Ingredients:

½ cup apple cider vinegar

4 pounds red jalapeno peppers, stems, seeds and ribs removed, chopped

10 garlic cloves, chopped

½ cup tomato paste

Juice of 1 orange zest

½ cup honey

2 tablespoons soy sauce

2 teaspoons salt

Directions:

Add vinegar, garlic, peppers, tomato paste, orange juice, honey, zest, soy sauce and salt to your Slow Cooker.

Stir and close lid.

Cook on LOW for 8 hours.

Use as needed!

Nutrition:

Calories:33;

Carbohydrates: 8g;

Protein: 12g;

Fat: 4g;

Sugar: 0.2g;

Sodium: 608mg;

Fiber: 0g

175. Tantalizing Mushroom Gravy

Preparation Time: 5 minutes

Cooking Time: 5-8 hours

Servings: 2

Ingredients: 1/3 cup water

1 cup button mushrooms, sliced

¾ cup low-fat buttermilk

1 medium onion, finely diced

2 garlic cloves, minced

2 tablespoons extra virgin olive oil

2 tablespoons all-purpose flour

1 tablespoon fresh rosemary, minced

Freshly ground black pepper

Directions: Add the listed ingredients to your Slow Cooker. Place lid and cook on LOW for 5-8 hours.

Serve warm and use as needed!

Nutrition: Calories:190;

Carbohydrates: 4g;

Protein: 2g; Fat: 6g;

Sugar: 1g; Sodium: 514mg;

Fiber: 0g

176. Everyday Vegetable Stock

Preparation Time: 5 minutes

Cooking Time: 8-12 hours

Servings: 4

Ingredients:

2 celery stalks (with leaves), quartered

4 ounces mushrooms, with stems

2 carrots, unpeeled and quartered

1 onion, unpeeled, quartered from pole to pole

1 garlic head, unpeeled, halved across middle

2 fresh thyme sprigs

10 peppercorns

½ teaspoon salt

Enough water to fill 3 quarters of Slow Cooker

Directions:

Add celery, mushrooms, onion, carrots, garlic, thyme, salt,

peppercorn and water to your Slow Cooker.

Stir and cover .

Cook on LOW for 8-12 hours.

Strain the stock through a fine mesh cloth/metal mesh and discard solids.

Use as needed.

Nutrition:

Calories:38;

Carbohydrates: 1g;

Protein: 0g;

Fat: 1.2g;

Sugar: 0g;

Sodium: 408mg;

Fiber: 1g

177. Grilled Chicken with Lemon and Fennel

Preparation Time: 5 minutes

Cooking Time: 25 minutes

Servings: 5

Ingredients:

2 cups chicken fillets, cut and skewed

1 large fennel bulb

2 garlic cloves

1 jar green olives

1 lemon

Directions:

Pre-heat your grill to medium-high.

Crush garlic cloves.

Take a bowl and add olive oil and season with sunflower seeds and pepper.

Coat chicken skewers with the marinade.

Transfer them under the grill and grill for 20 minutes, making sure to turn them halfway through until golden.

Zest half of the lemon and cut the other half into quarters.

Cut the fennel bulb into similarly sized segments.

Brush olive oil all over the garlic clove segments and cook for 3-5 minutes.

Chop them and add them to the bowl with the marinade.

Add lemon zest and olives.
Once the meat is ready, serve
with the vegetable mix.

Enjoy!

Nutrition:

Calories:649;

Carbohydrates: 15g;

Protein: 28g;

Fat: 6g;

Sugar: 2g;

Sodium: 354mg;

Fiber: 1.7g

178. Caramelized Pork Chops and Onion

Preparation Time: 5 minutes

Cooking Time: 40 minutes

Servings: 4

Ingredients:

4-pound chuck roast

4 ounces green Chili, chopped

2 tablespoons of chili powder

½ teaspoon of dried oregano

½ teaspoon of cumin, ground

2 garlic cloves, minced

Directions: Rub the chops
with a seasoning of 1 teaspoon
of pepper and 2 teaspoons of
sunflower seeds.

Take a skillet and place it over
medium heat, add oil and allow
the oil to heat up

Brown the seasoned chop both
sides. Add water and onion to
the skillet and cover, lower the
heat to low and simmer for 20
minutes. Turn the chops over
and season with more
sunflower seeds and pepper.
Cover and cook until the water
fully evaporates and the beer
shows a slightly brown texture.
Remove the chops and serve
with a topping of the
caramelized onion.

Serve and enjoy!

Nutrition: Calories:47;

Carbohydrates: 4g;

Protein: 0.5g; Fat: 4g;

Sugar: 1.3g; Sodium: 604mg;

Fiber: 0g

179. Hearty Pork Belly Casserole

Preparation Time: 5 minutes

Cooking Time: 25 minutes

Servings: 4

Ingredients:

8 pork belly slices, cut into small pieces

3 large onions, chopped

4 tablespoons lemon

Juice of 1 lemon

Seasoning as you needed

Directions:

Take a large pressure cooker and place it over medium heat.

Add onions and sweat them for 5 minutes.

Add pork belly slices and cook until the meat browns and onions become golden.

Cover with water and add honey, lemon zest, sunflower seeds, pepper, and close the pressure seal.

Pressure cook for 40 minutes.

Serve and enjoy with a garnish of fresh chopped parsley if you prefer.

Nutrition: Calories: 753 Fat: 41g Carbohydrates: 68g Protein: 30g

Nutrition:

Calories:753;

Carbohydrates: 23g;

Protein: 36g;

Fat: 4g;

Sugar: 0g;

Sodium: 312mg;

Fiber: 0g

180. Fascinating Spinach and Beef Meatballs

Preparation Time: 10 minutes

Cooking Time: 20 minutes

Servings: 4

Ingredients:

½ cup onion

4 garlic cloves

1 whole egg

¼ teaspoon oregano

Pepper as needed

1 pound lean ground beef

10 ounces spinach

Directions:

Preheat your oven to 375 degrees F.

Take a bowl and mix in the rest of the ingredients, and using your hands, roll into meatballs.

Transfer to a sheet tray and bake for 20 minutes.

Enjoy!

Nutrition:

Calories:200;

Carbohydrates: 5g;

Protein: 29g;

Fat: 3g;

Sugar: 3g;

Sodium: 514mg;

Fiber: 1g

181.   Juicy and Peppery Tenderloin

Preparation Time: 10 minutes

Cooking Time: 20 minutes

Servings: 4

Ingredients:

2 teaspoons sage, chopped

Sunflower seeds and pepper

2 1/2 pounds beef tenderloin

2 teaspoons thyme, chopped

2 garlic cloves, sliced

2 teaspoons rosemary, chopped

4 teaspoons olive oil

Directions:

Preheat your oven to 425 degrees F.

Take a small knife and cut incisions in the tenderloin; insert one slice of garlic into the incision.

Rub meat with oil.

Take a bowl and add sunflower seeds, sage, thyme, rosemary, pepper and mix well.

Rub the spice mix over tenderloin.

Put rubbed tenderloin into the roasting pan and bake for 10 minutes.

Lower temperature to 350 degrees F and cook for 20 minutes more until an internal thermometer reads 145 degrees F.

Transfer tenderloin to a cutting board and let sit for 15 minutes; slice into 20 pieces and enjoy!

Nutrition:

Calories:490;

Carbohydrates: 1g;

Protein: 24g;

Fat: 9g;

Sugar: 0g;

Sodium: 408mg;

Fiber: 1.7g

182. Healthy Avocado Beef Patties

Preparation Time: 15 minutes

Cooking Time: 10 minutes

Servings: 2

Ingredients:

1 pound 85% lean ground beef

1 small avocado, pitted and peeled

Fresh ground black pepper as needed

Directions:

Pre-heat and prepare your broiler to high.

Divide beef into two equal-sized patties.

Season the patties with pepper accordingly.

Broil the patties for 5 minutes per side.

Transfer the patties to a platter.

Slice avocado into strips and place them on top of the patties.

Serve and enjoy!

Nutrition:

Calories:560;

Carbohydrates: 9g;

Protein: 38g;

Fat: 16g;

Sugar: 0.2g;

Sodium: 254mg;

Fiber: 1g

183. Ravaging Beef Pot Roast

Preparation Time: 10 minutes

Cooking Time: 1hour 15 minutes

Servings: 4

Ingredients:

3 ½ pounds beef roast

4 ounces mushrooms, sliced

12 ounces beef stock

1-ounce onion soup mix

½ cup Italian dressing, low sodium, and low fat

Directions:

Take a bowl and add the stock, onion soup mix and Italian dressing.

Stir.

Put beef roast in pan.

Add mushrooms, stock mix to the pan and cover with foil.

Preheat your oven to 300 degrees F.

Bake for 1 hour and 15 minutes.

Let the roast cool.

Slice and serve.

Enjoy with the gravy on top!

Nutrition:

Calories:700;

Carbohydrates: 10g;

Protein: 46g;

Fat: 3g;

Sugar: 0.2g;

Sodium: 823mg;

Fiber: 1g

184. Lovely Faux Mac and Cheese

Preparation Time: 15 minutes

Cooking Time: 45 minutes

Servings: 4

Ingredients:

5 cups cauliflower florets

Sunflower seeds and pepper to taste

1 cup coconut almond milk

½ cup vegetable broth

2 tablespoons coconut flour, sifted

1 organic egg, beaten

1 cup cashew cheese

Directions:

Preheat your oven to 350 degrees F.

Season florets with sunflower seeds and steam until firm.

Place florets in a greased ovenproof dish.

Heat coconut almond milk over medium heat in a skillet, make sure to season the oil with sunflower seeds and pepper.

Stir in broth and add coconut flour to the mix, stir.

Cook until the sauce begins to bubble.

Remove heat and add beaten egg.

Pour the thick sauce over the cauliflower and mix in cheese.

Bake for 30-45 minutes.

Serve and enjoy!

Nutrition:

Calories:229;

Carbohydrates: 9g;

Protein: 15g;

Fat: 6g;

Sugar: 1.2g;

Sodium: 412mg;

Fiber: 0.7g

185. Chicken and Cabbage Platter

Preparation Time: 9 minutes

Cooking Time: 14 minutes

Servings: 2

Ingredients:

½ cup sliced onion

1 tablespoon sesame garlic-flavored oil

2 cups shredded Bok-Choy

1/2 cups fresh bean sprouts

1 1/2 stalks celery, chopped

1 ½ teaspoons minced garlic

1/2 teaspoon stevia

1/2 cup chicken broth

1 tablespoon coconut aminos

1/2 tablespoon freshly minced ginger

1/2 teaspoon arrowroot

2 boneless chicken breasts, cooked and sliced thinly

Directions:

Shred the cabbage with a knife. Slice onion and add to your platter alongside the rotisserie chicken.

Add a dollop of mayonnaise on top and drizzle olive oil over the cabbage.

Season with sunflower seeds and pepper according to your taste.

Enjoy!

Nutrition:

Calories:368;

Carbohydrates: 8g;

Protein: 42g;

Fat: 12g;

Sugar: 2.2g;

Sodium: 783mg;

Fiber: 0g

186.   Hearty Chicken Liver Stew

Preparation Time: 10 minutes

Cooking Time: 10 minutes

Servings: 0

Ingredients:

10 ounces chicken livers

1-ounce onion, chopped

2 ounces sour cream

1 tablespoon olive oil

Sunflower seeds to taste

Directions:

Take a pan and place it over medium heat.

Add oil and let it heat up.

Add onions and fry until just browned.

Add livers and season with sunflower seeds.

Cook until livers are half cooked.

Transfer the mix to a stew pot.

Add sour cream and cook for 20 minutes.

Serve and enjoy!

Nutrition:

Calories:146;

Carbohydrates: 5g;

Protein: 14g;

Fat: 9g;

Sugar: 0.5g;

Sodium: 254mg;

Fiber: 1.6g

Dessert Recipes

187. Delicious Lava Cake

Preparation Time: 15 minutes

Cooking Time: 20 minutes

Servings: 2

Ingredients

4 tablespoons of cocoa powder.

2 tablespoons of powdered swerve.

1/2 teaspoon of baking powder.

1/8 teaspoon of kosher salt to taste.

eggs.

tablespoons of heavy whipping cream.

2 teaspoons of pure vanilla extract.

Directions Preheat oven to 350 degrees F, grease a ramekin with non-stick cooking spray then set aside. Using a large mixing bowl, add in all the dry ingredients on the list then mix properly to combine until there are no more lumps.

In another mixing bowl, add in the eggs and beat. Add in other ingredients like the heavy cream and vanilla then mix everything to combine. Pour the egg mixture into the bowl containing the dry ingredients then mix everything properly to combine.

Pour the batter into the greased dish, place the dish into the preheated oven and bake the cake for about ten to fifteen minutes. Serve.

Nutrition: Calories:148;

Carbohydrates: 6.5g;

Protein: 16; Sugar: 2.2g;

Sodium: 252mg;

Fiber: 1g

188. Chocolate mousse cake

Preparation Time: 15 minutes

Cooking Time: 2hours 30 minutes

Servings: 12

Ingredients

Cake

1/2 cup of coconut flour.

eggs, separated.

1/2 cup of erythritol sweetener.

1/2 cup of unsalted butter.

1/2 teaspoon of baking powder.

1/3 cup of cocoa powder.

5 tablespoons of coconut milk.

Mousse

1.5 cups of whipping cream.

1.25 cups of chocolate chips.

3 tablespoons of rum which is optional.

Directions

Preheat the oven to 350F degrees F, place a parchment paper on a springform cake pan, grease properly then set aside. Using a small mixing bowl, add in the butter and sweetener then mix properly to combine. Add in the egg yolks and milk then mix again to combine.

Next, add in the flour, baking powder, and cocoa powder then mix again to combine, set aside. In another mixing bowl, add in the egg whites then whisk until it becomes stiff. Pour the egg white into the cake mixture then mix everything to combine.

Pour the mixture into the prepared pan, place the pan into the preheated oven and bake the cake for about thirty minutes until an inserted toothpick comes out clean, set aside to cool. For the mousse, melt the chocolate in a microwave for a few seconds then set aside.

Next, place the cream in a mixing bowl then whip until

there is a formation of stiff peaks. Pour the cream into the melted chocolate, add in the rum then stir everything to combine.

Spoon the prepared mousse over the cake, let the cake chill for about two hours to form up, slice and serve.

Nutrition:

Calories:428;

Carbohydrates: 6.5g;

Protein: 24g;

Fat: 35g;

Sugar: 2.2g;

Sodium: 654mg;

Fiber: 1g

189. Chocolate pie delis

Preparation Time: 30 minutes

Cooking Time: 15 minutes

Servings: 8

Ingredients

For the crust

2 cups of toasted almond flour.

8 tablespoons of melted butter.

2 tablespoons of unsweetened cocoa.

1 teaspoon of organic ground coffee.

1 teaspoon of vanilla extract.

8 drops of liquid stevia.

2-4 tablespoons of powdered monk fruit sweetener.

Filling

unces of cream cheese.

tablespoons of sour cream.

tablespoons of grass-fed butter.

tablespoon + 1 teaspoon of vanilla extract.

1/2 cup + 2 teaspoons of powdered monk fruit.

1/2 cup of unsweetened cocoa powder.

cup of heavy whipping cream.

1/8 teaspoon of almond extract.

8 drops of liquid stevia.

Directions

To make the crust, preheat the oven to 350 degrees F, grease a pie pan with coconut oil then set aside. Using a mixing bowl, add in the flour, butter, cocoa, ground coffee, vanilla extract, stevia, and monk fruit sweetener then mix everything properly to combine with a spatula.

Place the crust mixture into the greased pie pan, press out the mixture to evenly distribute in the pan, place the pan into the pleathered oven and bake the crust for about eighteen minutes, set aside.

For the pie, using a large mixing bowl, add in the cream cheese, butter, sour cream, 1 tablespoon of vanilla, 1/2 cup of powdered monk fruit, and cocoa powder then mix properly to combine. Use a hand mixer to mix again until the mixture becomes fluffy and combined.

Using another mixing bowl, add in the whipping cream, 2 teaspoons of monk fruit, 1 teaspoon of vanilla, almond extract, and stevia then mix with a hand mixer until peaks form. Pour the cream mixture into the bowl with the cocoa mixture then mix everything to combine.

Add the mixture into the prepared crust, then place the pie into the refrigerator to firm up. Slice the pie and serve.

Nutrition:

Calories:268;

Carbohydrates: 4.5g;

Protein: 2.4g;

Fat: 6.4g;

Sugar: 1.7g;

Sodium: 254mg;

Fiber: 2g

190.   Coffee Cake

Preparation Time: 40 minutes

Cooking Time: 20 minutes

Servings: 4

Ingredients

Coffee cake

3 cups of almond flour.

1/4 cup of stevia.

1/2 tablespoons of baking powder.

1/2 teaspoons of ground cinnamon.

teaspoon of sea salt to taste.

1/4 teaspoon of baking soda.

1/4 teaspoon of nutmeg.

1/2 cup (1 stick) of melted butter.

1 cup of sour cream.

2 eggs.

Streusel topping

2 cup of almond flour.

1/2 cup of coconut flour.

1/2 cup of stevia.

1/2 cup of pecans or walnuts.

1/2 cup (1 stick) sliced butter.

teaspoons of ground cinnamon.

1/4 teaspoon of sea salt to taste.

Directions

Preheat the oven to 350 degrees F, grease a cake pan with butter then set aside. For the topping, using a mixing bowl, add in the stevia, flours, pecan nuts, cinnamon, and salt to taste then mix to combine. Add in the sliced butter then mix until the mixture becomes a coarse crumb, set aside.

For the cake, mix the flour, stevia, spices, baking powder, baking soda, sea salt to taste then mix properly to combine. In another bowl, add in the melted butter, sour cream, and eggs then mix properly to combine. Pour the mixture into the bowl containing the flour mixture then mix everything to combine.

Place the batter into a springform pan, place the

topping over the cake batter, place the pan into the preheated oven and bake the cake for about forty-five minutes to one hour until the cake becomes brown in color and baked through.

Once baked, let the cake cool for a few minutes, slice, and serve.

Nutrition:

Calories:283;

Carbohydrates: 7.1g;

Protein: 5.9g;

Fat: 28.5g;

Sugar: 1g;

Sodium: 1254mg;

Fiber: 1g

191.   Delicious Brownies

Preparation Time: 10 minutes

Cooking Time: 20 minutes

Servings: 8

Ingredients

1/2 cup of almond flour.

1/4 cup of cocoa powder.

3/4 cup of erythritol.

1/2 teaspoon of baking powder.

tablespoon of instant coffee which is optional.

ablespoons of butter.

oz. of dark chocolate.

3 eggs.

1/2 teaspoon of vanilla extract which is optional.

Directions

Preheat the oven to 350 degrees F, place a parchment paper on a baking pan then grease properly with butter, set aside. Using a mixing bowl, add in the flour, cocoa powder, baking powder, erythritol, and coffee then whisk properly to combine. Place a skillet pan over medium heat, add in the chocolate and butter then melt for a few minutes.

Take the chocolate mixture out of the heat, add in the egg and vanilla then whisk properly to combine. Add in the flour mixture then mix again to combine. Pour the batter into the prepared baking pan, place the pan into the preheated oven and bake the brownies for about eighteen to twenty minutes until baked through. Once baked, let the brownies cool in the fridge for about thirty minutes to two hours, slice and serve.

Nutrition:

Calories:490;

Carbohydrates: 3g;

Protein: 2g;

Fat: 11g;

Sugar: 2.2g;

Sodium: 564mg;

Fiber: 0g

192. Chocolate chip cookies

Preparation Time: 10 minutes

Cooking Time: 12 minutes

Servings: 8

Ingredients

1 egg.

1/2 cup of Swerve sweetener.

1/3 cup of organic coconut oil.

1 teaspoon of pure vanilla extract.

1 1/2 cups of blanched almond flour.

1/2 teaspoon of baking soda.

1/4 teaspoon of sea salt to taste.

1/2 cup of dark chocolate chips.

Directions

Preheat the oven to 325 degrees F, place a parchment paper on a baking sheet then set aside. using a large mixing bowl, add in the egg and sweetener then whisk properly to combine. Add in the oil and vanilla then whisk again to combine. Add in the flour, baking soda, and salt to taste then mix properly to combine until there is a formation of a dough.

Next, fold in the chocolate chips, use a cookie scoop to form cookie shapes out of the dough then place them into the prepared baking sheet. Place the baking sheet into the preheated oven and bake the cookies for about ten to twelve minutes until they become light brown in color.

Once baked, let the cookies cool for a few minutes then serve.

Nutrition:

Calories:129;

Carbohydrates: 5g;

Protein: 1g;

Fat: 2g;

Sugar: 1.2g;

Sodium: 654mg; Fiber: 1g

193. Chocolate Mousse

Preparation Time: 10 minutes

Cooking Time: 0 minutes

Servings: 10

Ingredients

3 ounces of softened cream cheese.

1/2 cup of heavy cream.

1 teaspoon of vanilla extract.

1/4 cup of powdered Swerve.

2 tablespoons of cocoa powder.

1 pinch of salt to taste.

Directions

Using a large mixing bowl, add in the cream cheese then beat with an electric mixer until it becomes light and fluffy. Add in the heavy cream and vanilla extract then beat on a low setting. Add in the swerve, cocoa powder, and salt to taste then beat until everything is incorporated.

Mix again for about one to two minutes on a high setting until the mixture becomes light and fluffy. Serve.

Nutrition:

Calories:373;

Carbohydrates: 6.9g;

Protein: 8.4g;

Fat: 6.9g;

Sugar: 0g;

Sodium: 865mg;

Fiber: 2g

194.   Carrot Cake

Preparation Time: 35 minutes

Cooking Time: 15 minutes

Servings: 4

Ingredients

5 medium eggs.

7 oz. of melted butter.

3 tablespoons of low carb granulated sweetener.

2 teaspoons of vanilla.

3 cups of grated or shredded carrots.

1/2 cup of chopped walnuts.

1/2 cup of shredded and unsweetened coconut.

1 1/2 cups of almond flour.

1 teaspoon of ground cinnamon.

1 teaspoon of mixed spice.

2 teaspoons of baking powder.

Ginger which is optional.

Cream Cheese Frosting

7 oz. of cream cheese.

1 tablespoon of low carb granulated sweetener.

Directions

Using a large mixing bowl, add in the eggs, butter, sweetener, and vanilla then beat properly to combine. Add in other ingredients like the grated carrot, walnuts, and coconut then mix to combine. Add in the almond flour, spices, and baking powder then mix everything to combine.

Preheat the oven to 350 degrees F, place a parchment paper on a baking pan then set aside. pour the cake mixture into the baking pan, place the pan into the preheated oven and bake the cake for about forty to fifty minutes until an inserted toothpick comes out clean, set aside to cool.

To make the frosting, melt the cream cheese in a microwave for a few seconds then pour into a plate. add in the sweetener and lemon zest then mix properly to combine. Frost the cake as desired, slice and serve.

Nutrition:

Calories:321;

Carbohydrates: 6.5g;

Protein: 29.4g;

Fat: 2.6g;

Sugar: 2.3g;

Sodium: 965mg;

Fiber: 5g

195. Delicious Chocolare Cake

Preparation Time: 10 minutes

Cooking Time: 10 minutes

Servings: 8

Ingredients

1 1/2 cups of fine almond flour.

1/4 cup of cocoa powder.

2 tablespoons of Dutch cocoa.

2 1/4 teaspoon of baking powder.

1/2 teaspoon of salt to taste.

1/3 cup of almond milk.

3 eggs.

1/3 cup of granulated erythritol.

1 1/2 teaspoon of pure vanilla extract.

Directions

Preheat the oven to 350 degrees F, place a parchment paper on a baking pan then grease with non-stick cooking spray, set aside. Using a large mixing bowl, add in the flour, cocoa powder, Dutch cocoa, sweetener, and salt to taste then mix properly to combine.

In another mixing bowl, add in the eggs, vanilla extract, and milk the mix properly to combine. Pour the mixture into the bowl containing the flour then mix properly to combine. Pour the mixture into the prepared baking pan, smooth down with another parchment paper then place the pan into the preheated oven.

Bake the cake for about fourteen minutes until baked through. Frost as desired then serve.

Nutrition:

Calories:130;

Carbohydrates: 6g;

Protein: 17g;

Fat: 6g;

Sugar: 2.2g;

Sodium: 541mg;

Fiber: 3.4g

196.   Chocolate ice cream

Preparation Time: 35 minutes

Cooking Time: 2hours

Servings: 4

Ingredients

1 1/2 cups of heavy cream.

3/4 cups of unsweetened almond milk.

1/3 cup of dark cocoa powder.

1/3 cup of Swerve.

1/3 cup of xylitol.

3 large egg yolks.

2 ounces of unsweetened and chopped chocolate.

1/2 teaspoon of vanilla extract.

1/8 teaspoon of salt to taste.

Directions

Place a saucepan over medium heat, add in the cream, 1/2 cup of milk, cocoa powder, and sweeteners then cook while whisking until the mixture attains a temperature of 160 degrees F. Using a small mixing bowl, add in the eggs then whisk. Add in about a half cup of the cream mixture then whisk to combine.

Next, pour the yolk mixture into the saucepan then whisk to combine. Cook the mixture for a few minutes until it becomes thick and reaches 165 degrees F. don't forget to whisk as you cook, set aside. Add in the chopped chocolate, let the chocolate melt for about five minutes then mix properly until the mixture becomes smooth.

Place a bowl on an ice bath, pour the mixture into the bowl then let cool for a few minutes. Pour the mixture into a plastic bag, wrap tightly then refrigerate for about three hours. Next, add in the rest of the milk, vanilla extract, and salt to taste then whisk to combine. Pour the ice cream mixture into an ice cream maker then follow the instructions of a manufacturer. Serve.

Nutrition:

Calories:226;

Carbohydrates: 3.5g;

Protein: 6g;

Fat: 20.6g;

Sugar: 2.2g;

Sodium: 504mg;

Fiber: 3.6g

197.   Vanilla Ice Cream

Preparation Time: 30 minutes

Cooking Time: 0 minutes

Servings: 8

Ingredients

2 cups of heavy whipping cream.

1/2 cup of powdered erythritol.

1 pasteurized egg yolk.

1 tablespoon of vanilla extract.

Directions

Using a food processor or a high-speed blender, add in the

whipping cream, sweetener, yolk, and vanilla extract then blend until the mixture combines properly.

Pour the mixture into an ice cream maker and make the ice cream according to the directions of the manufacturer. Serve.

Nutrition:

Calories:205;

Carbohydrates: 4g;

Protein: 29.4g;

Fat: 0g;

Sugar: 2.6g;

Sodium: 486mg;

Fiber: 0g

198. Red Velvet Cupcakes

Preparation Time: 15 minutes

Cooking Time: 25 minutes

Servings: 8

Cupcake batter:

2 cups of almond flour.

2 tablespoons of Dutch cocoa.

3 tablespoons of butter.

1/3 cup of monk fruit/erythritol blend.

3 eggs.

1/2 cup of sour cream.

1/3 cup of buttermilk.

2 teaspoon of red food coloring.

1 teaspoon of baking powder

Icing

1/2 stick butter.

2 tablespoon of mascarpone cheese.

8 oz. of cream cheese.

1/4 cup of monk fruit sweetener.

1 teaspoon of vanilla.

Directions

Using a large mixing bowl, add in the flour, cocoa, and baking powder then mix properly to combine. In another mixing bowl, add in the butter, sweetener, and eggs then beat properly with a stand mixer.

Add in the sour cream, buttermilk, and red coloring then beat again to combine.

Next, pour the egg mixture into the bowl containing the flour mixture then stir everything to combine. Place parchment paper on a multi-well muffin tin, pour in the batter, place the muffin tin into an oven and bake at 350 degrees F for about twenty-five to thirty minutes until an inserted toothpick comes out clean, set aside to cool.

To make the icing, beat all its ingredients in a mixing bowl until the mixture becomes smooth. ice the cupcakes as desired then serve.

Nutrition: Calories:377;

Carbohydrates: 5.5g;

Protein: 7.4g; Fat: 24g;

Sugar: 2.2g;

Sodium: 345mg;

Fiber: 2.5g

199. Chocolate Milkshake

Preparation Time: 5 minutes

Cooking Time: 0 minutes

Servings: 1

Ingredients

1/2 cup of full-fat coconut milk or heavy cream.

1/2 medium and sliced avocado.

1-2 tablespoons of cacao powder.

1/2 teaspoon of vanilla extract.

Pink Himalayan salt to taste.

2-4 tablespoons of erythritol.

1/2 cup of ice.

Water as needed.

optional add-ins:

MCT oil

Hemp hearts

Collagen peptides

Mint extract or extract of choice

Directions

Using a food processor or a high-speed blender, add in all

the ingredients on the list (aside from the ice) alongside your chosen add ins then blend until the mixture becomes creamy and smooth. pour the mixture into a serving cup, add in the ice then serve.

Nutrition:

Calories:303;

Carbohydrates: 10.7g;

Protein: 3g;

Fat: 31g;

Sugar: 1.2g;

Sodium: 1234mg;

Fiber: 1.4g

200.   Chocolate Truffles

Preparation Time: 10 minutes

Cooking Time: 10 minutes

Servings: 16

Ingredients

9 oz. of sugar-free dark chocolate chips.

1/2 cup of heavy whipping cream or coconut milk.

1 teaspoon of cinnamon or sugar-free vanilla.

2 tablespoons of cacao powder for dusting.

Directions

Place a saucepan over medium heat, add in the cream and the cinnamon or vanilla then heat for a few minutes until it starts to simmer.

Place the chocolate in a mixing bowl, pour in the heated cream mixture then let sit for a few minutes until the chocolate dissolves, stir to combine.

Place the mixture into the refrigerator to chill for about two hours. Once chilled form small balls out of the mixture then roll in the cacao powder, serve.

Nutrition: Calories:190;

Carbohydrates: 2.5g;

Protein: 1.9g; Fat: 5g;

Sugar: 1.6g; Sodium: 476mg;

Fiber: 3.7g

Conclusion

It may seem daunting to turn to a ketogenic diet, but it does not have to be challenging. The attention will be on raising the carbohydrates while raising the meals & snacks ' fat and protein content. Carbs must be limited to enter and stay in a state of ketosis. Though some people can only get ketosis by consuming less than 20 g of carbs a day, others may be effective with a much high intake of carb. Typically speaking, the less the intake of carbohydrates, the easier it's to enter and remain in ketosis. That is why committing to keto-friendly meals and eliminating carbohydrate-rich products is the easiest way of losing weight on a keto diet. Among the most famous — and controversial— diets in recent memory to sweep the lifestyle scene is the keto diet.

veryone gradually gets older. It is an undeniable fact of life. But even though we are aging all of the time, we do not need to be old, not yet anyway. It is possible to be an active, vibrant woman at fifty and beyond if you make some smart choices and take care of yourself. And deciding to follow the keto way of life is the smartest choice you could have made. The keto diet isn't just good for weight loss, although that is probably its most important and noticeable feature. The keto diet gives so much more to your body while it is helping you to lose and then maintain your weight.

The keto diet will result in increased brain function and the ability to focus. The brain normally uses sugar to fuel its processes, but the consumption of sugar has its own problems. The brain can easily switch to using ketones for fuel and energy. Remember that ketones are the by-product of ketosis that makes you burn fat. And the keto diet was used by doctors to control seizures in patients long before medications were invented. The exact way this works is still not completely understood, but researchers believe it has something to do with the neurons stabilizing as excess sugar is removed from the diet and hormones are better regulated. Patients with Alzheimer's disease have been seen to have increased cognitive function and enhanced memory when they consume a keto diet. And these same changes in the chemical makeup of the brain can lead to fewer migraines overall and less severe migraines.

When the keto diet helps you to lose weight, it also helps you to reduce your risk of cardiovascular disease. These diseases include anything that pertains to the cardiovascular system, which means heart attacks, strokes, plaque formations, peripheral artery disease, blood clots, and high blood pressure. Plaque buildups, which are caused by excess weight and cholesterol, lead to a condition known as atherosclerosis. The plaque will gather in the arteries and form clogs that narrow the artery and restrict the flow of blood. The plaque is formed from fat cells, waste products, and calcium deposits that are found floating in the blood. When you lose weight and decrease the amount of fat and cholesterol in the body there will be less to accumulate in the arteries and the blood will naturally flow better with less restriction.

Being overweight can cause high blood pressure. When the doctor measures the force of your blood pressure as it moves through your arteries, he is measuring your blood pressure. If you are overweight your heart will need to push the blood harder to get it through the increased lengths of arteries it had to create in order to feed your cells. And if there is a buildup of plaque in the arteries then the heart will need to push the blood harder to get it past the blockage. This, in turn, creates thin spots in the arteries which is a good place for plaque to build up. Since this condition comes on gradually over the course of years as you slowly gain weight it gives off no immediate symptoms and that is why it is often referred to as the silent killer. Strokes and heart attacks are caused by unchecked high blood pressure.

The single most important way to control high blood pressure is to control your weight. You can't change the family history but you can control your weight and your lifestyle. Since high blood pressure is caused by the heart needing to work harder than the act reducing the strain on the heart will cause it to work less strenuously in bad ways. Losing weight and maintaining a healthy weight will ease the strain on your heart. If the blood pressure is not pumping too high then it will not cause weak spots in your arteries. If there are no weak spots then there is no place for plaque to collect. And if there is no excess fat or cholesterol in the blood there will be no plaque formations to collect in the blood.

A diet that is high in saturated fats is a risk factor for heart disease. While keto is a high-fat diet it is high in monounsaturated fats.

Polyunsaturated and monounsaturated fats are good for you while trans fats and saturated fats are not. Mono – and polyunsaturated fats are the good fats that are found in fatty fish like salmon and in certain plants like avocados, olives, and certain seeds and nuts that are all staples of the keto diet. Saturated fats and trans fats are found in breaded deep-fried foods, baked goods, processed foods, and pre-packaged snack foods like popcorn. When your doctor measures your LDL and HDL he also measures your level of triglycerides, which is a type of fat that is found floating in the bloodstream and that is responsible for elevating the risk of heart attacks, especially in women over fifty. Reducing the number of saturated fats and trans fats that you consume will automatically reduce the amounts of triglycerides floating in your blood. Inflammation is a part of life, especially for women over the age of fifty. There are good kinds of inflammation, such as when white blood cells rush to a particular body area to kill an infection. But mostly older women are plagued by the bad forms of inflammation which make your joints swell and cause early morning stiffness. Carrying too much weight on your body will cause inflammation and pain in the joints, especially in the lower part of the body where the weight-bearing joints like the knees and the hips are located. When a joint feels pain it sends a signal to the brain that there is a pain, and the body sends cells to combat that pain. The helper cells don't know there really isn't anything wrong but they come prepared to fight and this causes inflammation around the joint. One extra pound of excess weight will put four pounds of pressure on the knee joints. Losing weight will help to eliminate inflammation in the body. And cutting down on the intake of carbs will help to lessen the amount of inflammation in the body because carbs cause inflammation. Decreasing the inflammation in your body will also help to eliminate acne, eczema, arthritis, psoriasis, and irritable bowel syndrome.

Adopting the keto way of life will also help to eliminate problems with the kidneys and improve their function. Kidney stones and gout are caused mainly by the elevation of certain chemicals in the urine that helps to create uric acid which is what we eliminate in the bathroom. The excess consumption of carbohydrates and sugar will lead to a buildup of calcium and phosphorus in your urine. This buildup of excess chemicals can cause kidney stones and gout. When your ketones begin to raise the acid in your urine will briefly increase as your body begins to eliminate all of the waste products from the fats that are being metabolized, but after that, the level will decrease and will remain lower than before as long as you are on the keto diet.

This eating plan is low-carbon and high-fat and also can help you lose weight like crazy, but it also triggers extreme cravings, hormonal changes, mood swings, and is something profoundly unpleasant called "keto flu." The diet functions by cutting out carbohydrates and sugar, rapidly replenishing the body's energy reServings, and pushing it to find new sources of food that will be better for the nervous system and brain. The body begins producing ketones at a higher rate through eating a diet rich in the fats found naturally such as coconut oil, almonds, avocado & fatty fish.